Statistical Learning for Biomea. __

This book is for anyone who has biomedical data and needs to identify variables that predict an outcome, for two-group outcomes such as tumor/not tumor, survival/death, or response from treatment. Statistical learning machines are ideally suited to these types of prediction problems, especially if the variables being studied may not meet the assumptions of traditional techniques.

Learning machines come from the world of probability and computer science, but are not yet widely used in biomedical research. This introduction brings learning machine techniques to the biomedical world in an accessible way, explaining the underlying principles in nontechnical language and using extensive examples and figures. The authors connect these new methods to familiar techniques by showing how to use the learning machine models to generate smaller, more easily interpretable, traditional models.

Coverage includes single decision trees, multiple-tree techniques such as Random Forests™, neural nets, support vector machines, nearest neighbors, and boosting.

Practical Guides to Biostatistics and Epidemiology

Series advisors

Susan Ellenberg, *University of Pennsylvania School of Medicine*
Robert C. Elston, *Case Western Reserve University School of Medicine*
Brian Everitt, *Institute for Psychiatry, King's College London*
Frank Harrell, *Vanderbilt University Medical Center Tennessee*
Jos W.R. Twisk, *Vrije Universiteit Medical Centre, Amsterdam*

This series of short and practical but authoritative books is for biomedical researchers, clinical investigators, public health researchers, epidemiologists, and non-academic and consulting biostatisticians who work with data from biomedical and epidemiological and genetic studies. Some books explore a modern statistical method and its applications, others may focus on a particular disease or condition and the statistical techniques most commonly used in studying it.

The series is for people who use statistics to answer specific research questions. Books will explain the application of techniques, specifically the use of computational tools, and emphasize the interpretation of results, not the underlying mathematical and statistical theory.

Published in the series
Applied Multilevel Analysis, by **Jos W.R. Twisk**
Secondary Data Sources for Public Health, by **Sarah Boslaugh**
Survival Analysis for Epidemiologic and Medical Research, by **Steve Selvin**

Statistical Learning for Biomedical Data

James D. Malley
National Institutes of Health, Bethesda, MD

Karen G. Malley
Malley Research Programming, Inc., Rockville, MD

Sinisa Pajevic
National Institutes of Health, Bethesda, MD

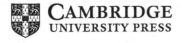

CAMBRIDGE
UNIVERSITY PRESS

CAMBRIDGE
UNIVERSITY PRESS

University Printing House, Cambridge CB2 8BS, United Kingdom

One Liberty Plaza, 20th Floor, New York, NY 10006, USA

477 Williamstown Road, Port Melbourne, VIC 3207, Australia

314-321, 3rd Floor, Plot 3, Splendor Forum, Jasola District Centre, New Delhi - 110025, India

79 Anson Road, #06-04/06, Singapore 079906

Cambridge University Press is part of the University of Cambridge.

It furthers the University's mission by disseminating knowledge in the pursuit of
education, learning and research at the highest international levels of excellence.

www.cambridge.org
Information on this title: www.cambridge.org/9780521875806

First published 2011

A catalogue record for this publication is available from the British Library

ISBN 978-0-521-87580-6 Hardback
ISBN 978-0-521-69909-9 Paperback

Cambridge University Press has no responsibility for the persistence or
accuracy of URLs for external or third-party internet websites referred to in
this publication, and does not guarantee that any content on such websites is,
or will remain, accurate or appropriate.

Contents

Preface		*page* xi
Acknowledgments		xii
Part I	**Introduction**	**1**
1	Prologue	3
	1.1 Machines that learn – some recent history	3
	1.2 Twenty canonical questions	7
	1.3 Outline of the book	9
	1.4 A comment about example datasets	11
	1.5 Software	12
	Note	13
2	The landscape of learning machines	**14**
	2.1 Introduction	14
	2.2 Types of data for learning machines	15
	2.3 Will that be supervised or unsupervised?	17
	2.4 An unsupervised example	18
	2.5 More lack of supervision – where are the parents?	20
	2.6 Engines, complex and primitive	20
	2.7 Model richness means what, exactly?	22
	2.8 Membership or probability of membership?	25
	2.9 A taxonomy of machines?	27
	2.10 A note of caution – one of many	30
	2.11 Highlights from the theory	30
	Notes	36
3	A mangle of machines	**41**
	3.1 Introduction	41

3.2	Linear regression	41
3.3	Logistic regression	42
3.4	Linear discriminant	43
3.5	Bayes classifiers – regular and naïve	45
3.6	Logic regression	47
3.7	k-Nearest neighbors	48
3.8	Support vector machines	50
3.9	Neural networks	53
3.10	Boosting	54
3.11	Evolutionary and genetic algorithms	55
	Notes	56
4	**Three examples and several machines**	**57**
4.1	Introduction	57
4.2	Simulated cholesterol data	58
4.3	Lupus data	61
4.4	Stroke data	62
4.5	Biomedical *means* unbalanced	63
4.6	Measures of machine performance	64
4.7	Linear analysis of cholesterol data	66
4.8	Nonlinear analysis of cholesterol data	67
4.9	Analysis of the lupus data	70
4.10	Analysis of the stroke data	75
4.11	Further analysis of the lupus and stroke data	79
	Notes	87
Part II	**A machine toolkit**	**89**
5	**Logistic regression**	**91**
5.1	Introduction	91
5.2	Inside and around the model	92
5.3	Interpreting the coefficients	93
5.4	Using logistic regression as a decision rule	94
5.5	Logistic regression applied to the cholesterol data	94
5.6	A cautionary note	98
5.7	Another cautionary note	101
5.8	Probability estimates and decision rules	102

5.9   Evaluating the goodness-of-fit of a logistic regression model   103

5.10 Calibrating a logistic regression   106

5.11 Beyond calibration   111

5.12 Logistic regression and reference models   113

Notes   115

6   A single decision tree   **118**

6.1   Introduction   118

6.2   Dropping down trees   118

6.3   Growing a tree   120

6.4   Selecting features, making splits   120

6.5   Good split, bad split   121

6.6   Finding good features for making splits   124

6.7   Misreading trees   125

6.8   Stopping and pruning rules   127

6.9   Using functions of the features   128

6.10 Unstable trees?   129

6.11 Variable importance – growing on trees?   132

6.12 Permuting for importance   134

6.13 The continuing mystery of trees   135

7   Random Forests – trees everywhere   **137**

7.1   Random Forests in less than five minutes   137

7.2   Random treks through the data   138

7.3   Random treks through the features   139

7.4   Walking through the forest   140

7.5   Weighted and unweighted voting   140

7.6   Finding subsets in the data using proximities   142

7.7   Applying Random Forests to the Stroke data   144

7.8   Random Forests in the universe of machines   151

Notes   153

Part III   **Analysis fundamentals**   **155**

8   Merely two variables   **157**

8.1   Introduction   157

8.2   Understanding correlations   158

8.3   Hazards of correlations   159

	8.4	Correlations big and small	163
	Notes		168
9	**More than two variables**		**171**
	9.1	Introduction	171
	9.2	Tiny problems, large consequences	172
	9.3	Mathematics to the rescue?	174
	9.4	Good models need not be unique	176
	9.5	Contexts and coefficients	179
	9.6	Interpreting and testing coefficients in models	181
	9.7	Merging models, pooling lists, ranking features	186
	Notes		190
10	**Resampling methods**		**198**
	10.1	Introduction	198
	10.2	The bootstrap	198
	10.3	When the bootstrap works	201
	10.4	When the bootstrap doesn't work	202
	10.5	Resampling from a single group in different ways	203
	10.6	Resampling from groups with unequal sizes	204
	10.7	Resampling from small datasets	206
	10.8	Permutation methods	207
	10.9	Still more on permutation methods	210
	Note		214
11	**Error analysis and model validation**		**215**
	11.1	Introduction	215
	11.2	Errors? What errors?	217
	11.3	Unbalanced data, unbalanced errors	218
	11.4	Error analysis for a single machine	219
	11.5	Cross-validation error estimation	222
	11.6	Cross-validation or cross-training?	224
	11.7	The leave-one-out method	226
	11.8	The out-of-bag method	227
	11.9	Intervals for error estimates for a single machine	228
	11.10	Tossing random coins into the abyss	230
	11.11	Error estimates for unbalanced data	232
	11.12	Confidence intervals for comparing error values	233

11.13	Other measures of machine accuracy	236
11.14	Benchmarking and winning the lottery	238
11.15	Error analysis for predicting continuous outcomes	239
	Notes	240

Part IV	**Machine strategies**	**245**
12	**Ensemble methods – let's take a vote**	**247**
12.1	Pools of machines	247
12.2	Weak correlation with outcome can be good enough	247
12.3	Model averaging	250
	Notes	254
13	**Summary and conclusions**	**255**
13.1	Where have we been?	255
13.2	So many machines	257
13.3	Binary decision or probability estimate?	259
13.4	Survival machines? Risk machines?	259
13.5	And where are we going?	260
	Appendix	263
	References	271
	Index	281

The color plate is situated between pages 244 and 245.

Preface

Statistical learning machines live at the triple-point of statistical data analysis, pure mathematics, and computer science. Learning machines form a still rapidly expanding family of technologies and strategies for analyzing an astonishing variety of data. Methods include pattern recognition, classification, and prediction, and the discovery of networks, hidden structure, or buried relationships. This book focuses on the problem of using biomedical data to classify subjects into just two groups. Connections are drawn to other topics that arise naturally in this setting, including how to find the most important predictors in the data, how to validate the results, how to compare different prediction models ("engines"), and how to combine models for better performance than any one model can give. While emphasis is placed on the core ideas and strategies, keeping mathematical gadgets in the background, we provide extensive plain-text translations of recent important mathematical and statistical results. Important learning machine topics that we don't discuss, but which are being studied actively in the research literature, are described in Chapter 13: Summary and conclusions.

Acknowledgments

This book evolved from a short lecture series at the invitation of Andreas Ziegler (University of Lübeck, Germany). Both he and Inke König (also at the University of Lübeck) live at the intersection of loyal friend, insightful analyst, and enabler of sound technical advances. We owe them our profound gratitude. Thank you both, Andreas and Inke.

Many others have also contributed significantly to this project. Collaborators at the National Institutes of Health have been numerous and helpful, over a long period of time. We especially single out: Joan Bailey-Wilson and Larry Brody (both at the National Human Genome Research Institute); Deanna Greenstein and Jens Wendland (both at the National Institute of Mental Health); Jack Yanovski, MD (National Institute for Child Health and Human Development); Michael Ward, MD, and Abhijit Dasgupta (both at the National Institute of Arthritis and Musculoskeletal and Skin Diseases); and John Tisdale (National Institute of Diabetes and Digestive and Kidney Diseases).

Other researchers, whose insight and support we also greatly appreciate, include: Luc Devroye (McGill University, Montreal); Gérard Biau (Université Pierre et Marie Curie, Paris); Carolin Stobl (Ludwig-Maximilians-Universität, München); Adele Cutler (Utah State University, Logan); Nathalie Japkowicz (Université d'Ottawa); Anna Jerebko (Siemens Healthcare, Germany); Jørgen Hilden (University of Copenhagen); and Paul Glasziou (University of Oxford).

We dedicate this book to Leo Breiman (1928–2005).

Part I

Introduction

Prologue

There is nothing like returning to a place that remains unchanged to find the ways in which you yourself have altered.

Nelson Mandela[1]

That is what learning is. You suddenly understand something you've understood all your life, but in a new way.

Doris Lessing

If we are always arriving and departing, it is also true that we are eternally anchored. One's destination is never a place but rather a new way of looking at things.

Henry Miller[2]

The only real voyage of discovery consists not in seeking new landscapes but in having new eyes.

Marcel Proust

1.1 Machines that learn – some recent history

Statistical learning machines arose as a branch of computer science. These intriguing computer-intensive methods are now being applied to extract useful knowledge from an increasingly wide variety of problems involving oceans of information, heterogeneous variables, and analytically recalcitrant data. Such problems have included:

- predicting fire severity in the US Pacific Northwest (Holden *et al.*, 2008);
- predicting rainfall in Northeastern Thailand (Ingsrisawang *et al.*, 2008);

---

[1] Nelson Mandela, *A Long Walk to Freedom* © Nelson Rolihlahla Mandela 1994. Reprinted by permission of Little, Brown and Company.
[2] Reproduced with permission of Curtis Brown Group Ltd, London on behalf of the Estate of Henry Miller © Henry Miller 1957. All rights reserved.

- handwriting recognition (Schölkopf and Smola, 2002);
- speech emotion classification (Casale *et al.*, 2008).

Learning machines have also been applied to biomedical problems, such as:

- colon cancer detection derived from 3-D virtual colonoscopies (Jerebko *et al.*, 2003, 2005);
- detecting differential gene expression in microarrays, for data that can involve more than a million single nucleotide polymorphisms (SNPs), in addition to clinical information, over several thousand patients (Díaz-Uriarte and Alvarez de Andrés, 2006);
- predicting short-term hospital survival in lupus patients (Ward *et al.*, 2006);
- finding the most predictive clinical or demographic features for patients having spinal arthritis (Ward *et al.*, 2009).

It is specifically toward this large class of clinical, biomedical, and biological problems that this book is directed. For example, for many important medical problems it is often the case that a large collection of heterogeneous data is available for each patient, including several forms of brain and neuroimaging data, a long stream of clinical values, such as blood pressure, age, cholesterol values, detailed patient histories, and much more. We will see that learning machines can be especially effective for analysis of such heterogeneous data where conventional parametric models are clearly not suitable, that is, where the standard assumptions for those models don't apply, can't easily be verified, or simply don't exist yet.

We alert the reader to the fact that there is a wide and growing range of terminology describing more or less the same area studied here. Prominent among these terms are *data mining, pattern recognition, knowledge discovery*, and our preferred choice, *machine learning*. Any such method, computer algorithm, or scheme can also be called a *prediction engine* if it claims to predict an outcome, discrete or continuous. From our perspective these mean the same thing.

In this framework, classical statistical procedures such as *logistic regression* or *linear regression* are simply classical examples of learning machines. These are parametric and model-based, as they ask the data to estimate some small number of coefficients (terms, parameters) in the model and often under specific assumptions about the probability distribution of the data (it's normally distributed, say). For example, given a set of features (clinical values, patient characteristics, numerous expensive measurements), a logistic regression model could be used to estimate the probability that a critically ill lupus patient will not survive the first 72 hours of an initial emergency hospital visit; see Ward *et al.* (2006).

On the other hand, most of the prediction engines we study are nonlinear and nonparametric models. The classic troika of data analysis assumptions – linearity, normality, and equal variance – is usually not invoked for learning machines. So, while the success of many statistical learning machine methods *does* rely on mathematical and statistical ideas (ranging from elementary to profound), the methods typically do not depend on, or derive their inspiration from, classical statistical outlooks.

That they often work as well as they do (or, notably, do not) is systematically studied under the heading of *probabilistic learning theory*; see Devroye *et al.* (1996). This is a rapidly developing area of research but this technical, foundational material is neither elementary nor easily summarized. Hence not even key conclusions are being widely taught to data analysts, and this has inhibited the adoption and understanding of learning machines. In this text we attempt to provide a summary, and also attempt to demystify another aspect of learning machines: the results of a given learning machine may be quite respectable in terms of low prediction error, say, but how the machine got to such a good prediction is often hard to sort out. Here, even a strong background in classical data analysis methods such as regression, correlation, and linear models, while a good thing in itself, may not be of much help, or more likely is just the beginning of understanding.

In dealing systematically with all these factors that have seemingly argued against broad acceptance of learning machines, we hope to keep the discussion relatively uncomplicated. Instead of making each page optically dense with equations we point the reader to some of the mathematical conclusions, but make an effort to keep the details out of sight. As such, the equations appear as heavily redacted and in translation from the original.

By traversing this territory we attempt to make another point: that working with statistical learning machines can push us to think about novel structures and functional connections in our data. This awareness is often counterintuitive, and familiar methods such as simple correlations, or the slightly more evolved partial correlations, are often not sufficient to pin down these deeper connections. We discuss these problems systematically in Part III: Analysis fundamentals.

Would that we could be as inventive and resourceful in our understanding as Nature is in setting the evidence before us each day.

There is another aspect of this journey that is important to mention up front. That is, many topics will reappear in different settings throughout this book. Among these are overfitting, interactions among predictor variables, measuring variable importances, classification vs. group probability membership, and resampling methods (such as the bootstrap, cross-validation). The reader can expect to uncover other repetitions. We think this reoccurrence of key topics is unavoidable and perhaps a good thing. How each topic arises and is, or is not, resolved in each instance, we hope will be reinforcing threads of the discussion.

Since the validity of the machine predictions do not typically derive mathematical comfort from standard parametric statistical methods (analysis of variance, correlations, regression analysis, normal distribution theory), we will also find that the predictions of statistical learning machines will push us to think carefully about the problem of *validating* those predictions.

There are two points here regarding validation. First, since the machines, these newer models, do not start from assumptions about the data – that it's normally distributed, say – a consequence is that devising procedures for testing the model is harder. Second, most of these procedures are reinforcing in their conclusions and are (often) nearly trivial to implement. Which is all to say that the work put into understanding unfamiliar connections in the data, and validating the machine predictions or estimations, is in itself a good thing and can have lasting scientific merit beyond the mechanics of the statistical learning methods we discuss.

Our first words of caution: we don't propose to locate any shining true model in the biological processes we discuss, nor claim that learning machines are, as a class of statistical procedures, uniquely wonderful (well, often wonderful, but not uniquely so). A statistical learning machine is a procedure that can potentially make good use of difficult data. And *if* it is shown to be effective in making a good prediction about a clinical process or outcome, it can lead us to refined understanding of that process: it can help us *learn* about the process.

Let's see what forms this learning can take . . .

1.2 Twenty canonical questions

Some highlights of this textbook, in the form of key questions, are presented. Some of these questions arise naturally in classical statistical analysis, and some arise specifically when using learning machines. Some of the questions are very open-ended, having multiple answers, some are themselves compound questions, while Question 20 is a trick question. Citations to chapters and sections in the book that provide solutions and discussions are given for each of the *Twenty Canonical Questions*:

(1) Are there any over-arching insights as to why (or when) one learning machine or method might work, or when it might not?

(Section 2.11)

(2) How do we conduct robust selection of the most predictive features, and how do we compare different lists of important features?

(Sections 6.6, 7.3, 9.7)

(3) How do we generate a simple, smaller, more interpretable model given a well fitting but much larger one that fits the data very well? That is, how do we move from an inscrutable, but highly predictive learning machine to a tiny, familiar kind of model? How do we move from an efficient black box to a simple open book?

(Section 5.12)

(4) Why does the use of a very large number of features, say 500K genetic expression values, or a million SNPs, very likely lead to massive overfitting? What exactly is overfitting and why is it a bad thing? How is it possible to do *any* data analysis when we are given 550,009 features (or, 1.2 million features) and only 132 subjects?

(Sections 2.6, 7.8)

(5) Related to (4), how do we deal with the fact that a very large feature list (500K SNPs) may also nicely predict entirely random (permuted) outcomes of the original data; how can we evaluate any feature selection in this situation?

(Sections 6.12, 10.8, 11.10)

(6) How do we interpret or define interactions in a model? What are the unforeseen, or the unwanted consequences of introducing interactions?

(Section 5.6)

(7) How should we do prediction error analysis, and get means or variances of those error estimates, for any single machine?

(Section 11.4)

(8) Related to (7), given that the predictions made by a pair of machines on each subject are correlated, how do we construct error estimate comparisons for the two machines?

(Section 11.12)

(9) Since unbalanced groups are a routine in biology, for example with 25 patients and 250 controls, what are the hazards and remedies?

(Sections 4.5, 10.6, 11.11)

(10) Can data consisting of a circle of red dots (one group) inside an outer circle of green dots (a second group) ever derive from a biologically relevant event? What does this say about simulated data?

(Section 2.11)

(11) How much data do we need in order to state that we have a good model and error estimates? Can classical statistics help with determining sample sizes for obtaining good models with learning machines, given that learning machines are often nonparametric and nonlinear?

(Section 2.11)

(12) It is common that features are quite entangled, having high-order correlation structure among themselves. Dropping features that correlated with each other can be quite mistaken. Why is that? How can very weak predictors, acting jointly, still be highly predictive when acting together?

(Chapter 9)

(13) Given that several models can look very different but lead to nearly identical predictions, does it matter which model is chosen in the end, or, is it necessary to choose any single model?

(Sections 9.4, 12.3)

(14) Closely related to (13), distinct learning machines, and statistical models in general, can be combined into a single, larger and often better model, so what combining methods are mathematically known to be better than others?

(Chapter 12)

(15) How do we estimate the probability of any single subject being in one group or another, rather than making a pure (0,1) prediction: "Doctor, you say I will

probably survive five years, but do I have a 58% chance of survival or an 85% chance?"

(Section 2.8)

(16) What to do with missing data occurring in 3% of a 500K SNP dataset? In 15.4% of the data? Must we always discard cases having missing bits here and there? Can we fill in the missing bits and still get to sound inference about the underlying biology?

(Section 7.8)

(17) How can a learning machine be used to detect – or define – biologically or clinically important subsets?

(Section 2.3)

(18) Suppose we want to make predictions for continuous outcomes, like temperature. Can learning machines help here, too?

(Section 2.2)

(19) How is it that using parts of a good composite clinical score can be more predictive than the score itself?

(Sections 4.3, 6.9)

(20) What are the really clever methods that work really well on *all* data?

(Sections 2.11, 11.14)

1.3 Outline of the book

Given the varied statistical or mathematical background the reader may have, and the relative novelty of learning machine methods, we divide the book into four parts.

Part I Introduction

A survey of the landscape of statistical learning machines is given, followed by a more detailed discussion of some specific machines. Then, we offer a chapter in which examples are given applying several learning machines to three datasets. These datasets include a simple computer-generated one that is still indicative of real-world data, one from published work on clinical predictions for lupus patients, and another also from published work related to a large study of stroke patient functional outcomes.

Part II A machine toolkit

Here we discuss three machines: logistic regression, decision trees, and Random Forests™. Logistic regression is a basic tool in biomedical data analysis, though usually not thought of as a learning machine. It is a parametric prediction scheme, and can give us a small, usually well-understood reference model. Single decision trees are but one instance of a very primitive learning machine, devices that often do surprisingly well, and yet also might not do so well, depending on the data structure, sample size, and more. We then discuss Random Forests, which as the name suggests are built from many (many!) single decision trees. Since its introduction by Leo Breiman and Adele Cutler (Breiman, 2004), it now has its own growing literature showing how it can be improved upon, and how it might not succeed. It also has two new and important incarnations, *Random Jungles* and *Conditional Inference Forests*; see Note 1. Random Forests is guaranteed to be good (under certain reasonable assumptions, according to theory), and can predict (estimate) continuous outcomes as well. Of course, as we will often point out, many other machines may do much better, or just as well, and the practical equivalence of various machines is a conclusion we usually see when there is at least a moderately strong signal in the data.

Part III Analysis fundamentals

No special statistical or mathematical or computer programming maturity is strictly required for this book. We assume the reader's statistical portfolio contains only some awareness of *correlations*, *regression analysis*, and *analysis of variance*. Very good reviews and discussions of these topics can be found, for example, in Agresti and Franklin (2009), Glantz (2002), Sprent and Smeeton (2001), and of course in many other excellent texts. However, we will also include some of the basics about correlation and regression, and offer a full discussion of the problems with both.

Given these analysis basics, we assert that statistical learning machines can push us toward new and unexpected appreciation of how data works and how structure can reveal itself. The Twenty Canonical Questions point in this direction, and as well, crafting the right question can be better than offering a simple answer.

We next discuss the problem of error analysis: estimates of how well a machine is doing. Finally, we address the problem of evaluating the predictive accuracy of two machines, by seeing how they do on each case (subject), one at a time. It is essential to witness that these outcomes on each case (subject) will generate a pair of results, and typically these will be correlated. Therefore, confidence intervals of the difference in error rates need to include this non-independence. While often overlooked in some technical studies of learning machines, this subject has recently (Tango, 1998, 1999, 2000; Newcombe, 1998a–c) been thoroughly upgraded in the statistical literature, and newer methods have demonstrated remarkable improvements over very classical methods. These improved methods, and the need for the improvements, are covered in Chapter 10.

Part IV Machine strategies

The final section of this book outlines a specific, practical strategy: use a learning machine for intensive, thorough processing of the data, and then if the error values seem promising, proceed using some subset of the features in a much smaller, more familiar model, such as logistic regression. Often the initial choice of learning machine (for example, a support vector machine instead of a Random Forest) is not too critical, if there is significant signal in the data, but there are important exceptions. And the choice of a small, interpretable model is not so important either, given a central interest in predictive accuracy. That is, as mentioned above and as discussed frequently below, if any good signal is present in the data then most learning machines will find it, and then many smaller models will fit equally well. There are many paths through the wilderness of validation. The important point is that a learning machine is only a single, initial element in thorough data analysis.

1.4 A comment about example datasets

As mentioned above, we study three biomedical datasets in Chapter 4. One of these, *Cholesterol*, is a simulated dataset, based on two measures of serum cholesterol. The second example, the *Lupus* study, appeared in a published collaboration (Ward *et al.*, 2006). The third example, the large *Stroke* study, also appeared in a published collaboration (König *et al.*, 2007, 2008). The stroke data was a multi-center study collected in two groups, allowing us the rare luxury of being able to systematically compare predictions made for each using the other.

In making these choices we generally refrained from directing the reader to listings of published data analyses using learning machines, or to public sites for machine learning data analysis. In our experience much of this published data is too clean, nicely structured, and beautifully manicured, and thus may not be similar to what you routinely encounter. Another thought here is that datasets are often used to merchandise one method over all others, but we know that such benchmarking is provably doomed: see item (3) in Section 2.11, and also Chapter 10. Of course, the subject-matter problems to which this public data points are all important, but they seem to us not sufficiently messy and hence not typical of what we encounter in biomedical data analysis.

More on datasets is given in Appendix A1.

1.5 Software

Computer code and related software for most of the statistical learning machines we discuss is freely available on the Web, in a variety of forms. All data were analyzed using one of several computer methods.

These included PROC LOGISTIC in SAS® version 9.1.3 and PROC IML code, macro %GOFLOGIT, using SAS® version 8.2.

For many of the simpler machines we implemented our own and used the code with MatLab®, but we also used R code (for Random Forests), C code (for SVMLight), and precompiled executables (for boosting), all ported into MatLab.

The R library (available online) is a standard source for such code and continues to evolve as new, faster, better versions of the procedures are developed in R. We provide a list of websites that lead the user to existing code, and point the reader to websites that deal with machine-learning issues. Making contact with the problem of intellectual advocacy, and the related problem of merchandising and promoting new code as mercantile enterprises, we caution the reader that many sites are too often organized for a quite specific reason: to promote the methods presented at the site.

Understandably some of these sites may not feel obligated to discuss how those methods may be less than optimal, how they might utterly fail, or how they compare rigorously with other learning machine methods, or even with simpler classical methods. We hope to provide tools for the reader to make such comparisons.

More on the code used in this text is given in Appendix A2.

Note

(1) *Random Jungles* was developed by Daniel F. Schwarz in 2006; go to randomjungle.com. *Conditional Inference Forests* was developed by Hothorn *et al.* (2006).

The landscape of learning machines

To give an idea of this rapidity, we need only mention that Mr. Babbage believes he can, by his engine, form the product of two numbers, each containing twenty figures, in three minutes. ... Now, admitting that such an engine can be constructed, it may be inquired: what will be its utility?

Ada Augusta, Daughter of Lord Byron, Countess of Lovelace (1842)

2.1 Introduction

In this chapter we outline general themes and ideas related to statistical learning machines. We frame the subject and some of its important analytic processes. Chapter 3 will discuss specific learning machines, with brief discussions of their individual advantages and disadvantages; see Note 1.

Readers wishing to travel a more direct path could consider skipping this chapter, going right to Chapter 3, and then straight on to Chapter 4, where many of the machines are put through their paces on three examples. However, a direct path, free of the context provided by this chapter, may leave the novice disoriented. This is because the geology of machine learning is not a single tectonic plate and is more a vast, still-expanding archipelago, with many separated islands of insight and research, some connected, some not.

Throughout this text we will frequently be quoting, or attempting to translate for the reader, from a wonderful but technically very advanced book, Devroye *et al.* (1996). This text is magisterial, huge – 635 pages! – dense and highly articulate. Going forward, we will use the abbreviation *DGL*.

Let's begin. In this book we focus on the problems of *prediction* and *classification* for groups of subjects, where it is assumed that the outcome, the status, for each subject is known explicitly. *Outcome* here means group membership {colon cancer, no colon cancer}, and *classification* means declaring group membership. For us *prediction* usually means classification, but more generally it can also mean estimating some continuous outcome {extent of spinal curvature}.

There is a breath-taking range of terminology used for describing more or less the same area studied here. Prominent among these terms are *data mining, pattern recognition, knowledge discovery*, and our preferred choice, *machine learning*. From our perspective these mean the same thing. Rather than attempt a semiotic or syntatic disection of these many terms, we simply delcare that any computer program whose intent, given data, is classification or estimation, is a learning machine. Also, we use as equivalent the terms *learning machine* and *classification scheme*, and often more colorfully: *prediction engine*; see Note 2.

There are a number of important areas of machine learning that are not discussed in this text. This growing list is discussed at the end of the book, Chapter 13, and includes prediction of survival, estimation of the probability of group membership, dependent data, and more. The list also includes prediction for continuous outcomes (the *regression problem*), a deep and varied topic in itself, and addressed in the text by Györfi *et al.* (2002). This text is just as long as *DGL* (647 pages!) and just as beautifully written. As a companion to both DGL and Györfi *et al.*, we can recommend Devroye and Lugosi (2001); and of course read Vapnik (2000), who was one of the founders of modern machine learning theory.

The larger point of all these texts and the research surrounding their results is that classical statistical methods can often be effectively replaced with fully nonparametric combinatorial methods. This subject is nontrivial, beautiful, and ultimately surprisingly practical.

2.2 Types of data for learning machines

Regarding what data might be suitable for the prediction problem of interest, we strongly encourage the reader to set aside conventional views of types of data allowed, limits on the number of features, and standard statistical modeling assumptions. Nearly all of the learning machines we describe are, *exactly by construction*, designed to work with data having arbitrary structure or type. Loosely speaking, the statistical learning machines studied here are, for the most part, massively nonparametric. More precisely, apart from an important exception (the naïve Bayes machine; see Chapter 3), we make absolutely no assumptions concerning the joint statistical distribution of the data; see Note 3.

This is an essential property of learning machines as we study them here, and some reformatting of belief concerning these aspects of data analysis is likely to be involved. The measurements themselves can be any combination of continuous or discrete, and the list of measurements can number in the millions. Indeed, regarding the number of measurements involved, some learning machines energetically introduce new functions of the original measurements. *Support vector machines* are of this type, as is the *logic regression* method. And the classifications (predictions) made by one or more learning machines can be creatively recycled and used as new measurements for input (features) to other machines. We support recycling. This is discussed in Chapter 5 (Logistic regression) and in Chapter 12 (Ensemble methods).

Given these preliminaries, the basic elements of our data are the *subject* and the *measurements* made on that subject. *Measurements*, for us, consist of two parts: (i) a list of *predictors* (features, attributes, categories, rates, assignments) and (ii) an associated *outcome* (result, category) for that subject or instance.

In the statistics literature these two parts are commonly called the independent and dependent variables, respectively. We will use the terms predictors, features, attributes, variables, etc. interchangeably to mean *measurements*. As noted above, some of these measurements themselves might be "outcomes" from tests, procedures, or even predictions made by other learning machines.

Extensions of learning machines to outcomes that have more than a binary list of possible results, say having group identification among four groups of tumor cell types, are becoming possible for many machines and under rapid development; see for example Archer and Mas (2009). The program Random Forests and the family of support vector machines, for example, have both been extended in this direction, and websites devoted to any one method generally announce these advances. However, we do not consider in detail here these important, newer inventions.

Also, not considered here and equally an important area of research is the situation where the outcome variable is itself a *list* of outcomes, for example {temperature, height, weight} or {thousands of genetic products or results}. Such data arises naturally in the study of gene expression transcripts, which can number in the tens of thousands, and for each such list there may be associated a very long collection of measurements: the values for each of 500,000 SNPs collected for each subject in a study of childhood-onset schizophrenia.

Let's now assume data has been collected on a group of subjects, where this data – patient attributes – might include patient history, clinical measurements, genetic data, neuroimaging data, and much more. And for each such collection of measurements on the subject we want to predict an outcome {tumor, not tumor} or {extent of severity of spinal arthritis}. In the machine-learning community these problems are described as examples of *supervised learning*, since the group membership is known for each subject – and the machine is then given a structured, supervised task. There is also an important branch of learning machines called *unsupervised learning* . . .

2.3 Will that be supervised or unsupervised?

We introduced above the term *supervised learning* to describe a learning machine that makes predictions, either for the status {tumor, no tumor} of a subject, or for some continuous value {total cholesterol} related to that subject. To help refine our understanding of just what it is that learning machines can do, we take a short tour of *unsupervised learning*; see Note 4.

This tour will also put on view the different uses possible for a given supervised learning machine. For example, we may find that beginning with a supervised learning approach we can, using unsupervised methods, uncover hidden structure in the data, or the measurements themselves, or both. These apparent findings can then, in turn, be studied more systematically using supervised methods. We still support recycling.

A fundamental example of *unsupervised learning* is the activity of *clustering*. Briefly, this is the attempt to organize the subjects into self-similar, more homogeneous, smaller subgroups. These new alternative groupings may or may not be related to the original groupings (status) of the subjects, and new interconnections can be uncovered in the data. For example, some subsets of tumor patients might seem, on closer inspection, to be more similar to normal subjects, with the remaining tumor patients quite different from that apparent subset *and* from the normal subjects. The notion of similarity here is the key working hypothesis; see *multidimensional scaling* below. There is a universe of possibility in this quiet and unassuming term: similarity.

Also under the heading of unsupervised learning is the process of finding structure in the measurements themselves. Here the task is finding relationships within and among the measurements on the subjects, with less emphasis on any outcomes or labels for the subjects. And given labels this search can be refined: the list of most predictive measurements for *this* subgroup seems quite different from the list relating to this *other* subgroup, so, why is that? Why are the connections between these basic clinical measurements different in these subgroups? Do these differential protein expression levels in this tumor subgroup tell us anything about the disease process itself? Are different metabolic pathways operating within the tumor group as opposed to the normal group, or to the other tumor subgroups? For these problems a different version of proximity is needed.

These are important questions not necessarily driven by the supervised learning, pure prediction problem, but subsequent to, arising after, the pure prediction problem. They can lead to important follow-up projects: what makes these patients, these variables, different? Can we use the data to make predictions specifically for these subgroups? These next-step questions are examples of recycling, which we support even now.

As mentioned above, in this book we will not focus very much on unsupervised learning, but for one important exception, that of *multidimensional scaling*. It can help us identify significant subgroups of patients, and subsets of variables ...

2.4 An unsupervised example

Multidimensional scaling is a collection of mathematical maneuvers that can be understood as unsupervised learning schemes. It is a corpus of techniques for transforming the data to reduce the possibly very high dimensionality of the problem, that is, to strip away inessential aspects of the data and reveal interior structure. Such transformations begin with a user-specified definition of a "distance" between the subjects and proceed to user-specified reductions that retain most of the original distance for each pair of subjects.

Technically it has a significant overlap with methods of *principal components analysis*; see Note 4.

The paragraph above will benefit from unpacking, so here is a specific instance of *multidimensional scaling*, one connected with a supervised machine. Suppose a classification scheme (learning machine) manages to partition (segment) all the data into small boxes, and places two subjects in the same box. A simple version of this could be the data box given by all those subjects with {height in the range 1.5 to 2.0 m, and weight in the range 68 to 77 kg}. Any two subjects in this box might belong to different groups (one being a cancer patient, the other a normal control). The boxes could in fact be defined by a long sequence of binary choices or splits in the data: those subjects with {high value on Test Marker 1, low value on Test Marker 2, and mid-level value on Test Marker 3}, and so on. Now, the occurrence of a pair of subjects falling into the same box, after the binary or even more complex sifting done by the machine, can be considered a measure of similarity or *proximity*, as defined by *this* learning machine. It suggests that the two subjects have something clinically in common, something not noticed as the data was collected, some important clinical aspect apart from their clinical status {cancer, no cancer}.

Next, consider making many such assignments of the subjects into boxes. This could arise from multiple applications of the same learning machine on slightly different copies of the data, or from multiple different machines that each lead to box assignments. For each pair of subjects we can calculate the fraction of times they appear in the same box across the many methods. Subjects appearing often together in this way, in this machine, suggest a higher proximity than those rarely appearing together.

Sorting all the subjects into small boxes and assigning proximities to every pair of subjects generates a large array (technically, a matrix) of proximities. Next, mathematically sophisticated transformations of this array then hold some promise for disaggregating the data, for identifying subsets, subgroups of patients worthy of clinical interest. In fact, there is a very large and still-growing library of possible distance measures and possible transformations; see Cox and Cox (2001), Borg and Groenen (2005).

Whether or not clustering into novel subgroups, as described above, using a specific user-defined notion of distance, is *biomedically* meaningful is an object of some contention in the literature: be prepared to defend any clinical subsets obtained from this effort at unsupervised learning, particularly the proximity measure underlying it; see Chapter 12.

2.5 More lack of supervision – where are the parents?

Other examples of unsupervised learning include the discovery of associations in the measurements, linkages, and relationships in these values. In Chapter 11 we discuss the challenge of grouping or clustering features and variables (rather than subjects). Specifically, how certain genes cooperate in a narrowly framed clinical setting can suggest metabolic or signaling pathways that in turn can lead to better understanding of the disease process. Or, quite unexpectedly and often happily, novel linkages can point to a biological overlap with other, but not clearly similar, disease processes. In both of these two instances it may therefore be possible to refine our original analysis (prediction) or refine our understanding of the basic disease process itself.

More formally, it is our belief that statistical learning which can be most rigorously validated takes place under a supervised approach: to make progress we need a target function or figure of merit (status, group membership, patient outcome) that has well-understood biological or clinical consequences. And it continues to be a challenge to transmute analytical suggestions made under unsupervised or casual learning about associations, and relationships among the measurements, into well-framed, validated inferences. But we also find that the results of a supervised approach can in turn be interrogated productively using an unsupervised scheme. Equally, it is a challenge to pull apart clinically important subgroups in the data. We can state this in the form of more Canonical Questions, similar to those listed in Chapter 1. How do we evaluate the overlap of two signaling or metabolic networks? How do we evaluate a scheme of associations detected in and among the measurements? How do we estimate the overlap of two clusters or subgroups in our data, or determine the clinical significance of the overlap?

2.6 Engines, complex and primitive

We have discussed supervised and unsupervised machines, and also parametric and nonparametric methods. There is another axis about which learning machines may be arranged. It is often the case that a learning machine can do very well on a dataset, in fact, suspiciously too well, and this identifies the problem of *overfitting*. Here the prediction engine does very nicely for the data we collected last week, but does really poorly on the new data we trained in on last week. Or, more worrisome, the engine has phenomenal accuracy on today's data but we're (correctly) worried that it might not do nearly so well for the next patient coming to the clinic.

One broad class of procedures for dealing with this problem is as follows: apply a very flexible, adaptive engine to the data, but somehow restrict its activity, its performance, on the data. We realize this seems deeply counterintuitive: why start with a flexible, highly adaptable method and then constrain it?

One answer is that a prediction engine can be too adaptable, and will not make allowances for the random variation that is part of any dataset. Indeed, most learning machines we discuss are applied to data for which we have exactly no built-in, *a priori* notion of the underlying statistical distribution. Learning machines therefore usually do not see the data in probability terms. Hence, given new data having this same random, but still unknown variation, a machine will necessarily do less well unless certain precautions are taken.

One approach to dealing with this problem, of doing very well on today's data and not very well on tomorrow's data, is to constrain the model, to limit its complexity. This can mean simply restricting the coefficients in the model in a clearly defined way. Fitting a straight line to the data is a restricted form of fitting a quadratic or cubic curve through the data. So, whereas a quadratic curve can be drawn through any three points in the plane – thus fitting those data points perfectly, indeed overfitting those points – a straight line is not so adaptable, but may better allow for random variation in the data.

In this approach the constraints are not usually data-dependent, that is, things needing estimation from the data, though in principle they could be. For example, a simple penalty or constraint in a linear model might be that {all true but unknown coefficients should be positive} and usually as well {all the estimated values for these coefficients should be positive}. Another kind of constraint is this: the sum of the absolute values of all the coefficients cannot be larger than some constant, where this bound is selected by the data analyst. This last method is the so-called *lasso*, now with numerous variants – see Tibshirani (1996), Ghosh and Chinnaiyan (2005), Ma and Huang (2008), Hastie *et al.* (2009).

It is important to see that the methods by which the parameters in any prediction engine or model are constrained or penalized can be quite different and have distinctly different results. Indeed, engines and statistical models generally, having different constraints, should be expected to make different predictions for the same subject. In any case, a constrained model that does only moderately well on today's data is attempting to allow for the underlying variability of the data in its predictions and hence make better statements about tomorrow's data. Otherwise stated, an infinitely rich, supremely flexible model, or family of models, probably will not generalize.

How to balance these different goals is an area of much active research. Part of the problem is deciding how we should best evaluate the relative merits of any sets of constraints. They can, for example, be considered under the rubric of methods for assigning numbers to any model's informativeness. For example, with the more familiar models such as those in linear regression and curve fitting, we can count the number of parameters (coefficients to be estimated) in the model and combine that value with an estimate of the goodness-of-fit for the model. This leads to summary information measures such as the *Akaike information criterion* (AIC), the *Bayesian information criterion* (BIC), and numerous variants. These methods usually require introducing the *likelihood function*; see DGL (chapter 15), Harrell (2001, chapter 9), Claeskens and Hjort (2008), Severini (2000). Again, in the universe of nonparametric methods, that universe in which most learning machines live, we don't assume that a probability distribution is available for the data, so we can't write down a likelihood function as a first step for parameter estimation and model evaluation.

Another practical problem regarding the use of parameter specifications for model richness or complexity is that many learning machines have either exactly zero parameters to be estimated, or, an infinite continuum of them. For example, a k-nearest-neighbor machine (see Section 3.7) has exactly zero parameters to be estimated, while a single classification tree (see Chapter 5) has an arbitrarily large number of "parameters."

2.7 Model richness means what, exactly?

This section is fairly heavy going technically, but we urge the reader to persist as far as possible, or make repeated efforts through the thicket.

An alternative, precise technical definition of the machine adaptability, or *model richness*, is the notion of *Vapnik–Chernovenkis (VC) dimension*. A precise and sophisticated notion of model richness was developed in the 1970s by Vapnik, Chernovenkis and co-workers; see DGL (section 12.4). This approach leads to some of the most profound generalizations of fundamental results in mathematical statistics. It stands as a beacon in the galaxy for all machine learners. And important practical facts about learning machines can be derived using the VC dimension. For example, it provides specific practical guidance on how to tune certain very good machines for any given sample size. It tells us when a family of learning machines will necessarily overfit any given dataset, so model penalties or parameter constraints would be required.

The starting point for this topic is the idea that a particularly rich family of functions (models, class of prediction engines, learning machines) should be good at separating out from a random collection of data points, any *subset* of the random points. Every class of functions (models, etc.) has a specific richness value, the VC dimension specifying how successful the class is at this separation problem. Prediction engines can then be graded in terms of richness, where presumably richer is better. If a class of functions is able to separate out *every* subset of a given set of points, then it is, most colorfully, said to *shatter* that set of points. The VC dimension for a family of prediction engines (classifiers, models) can, in principle, then be used to provide an upper bound on the large sample error made by any member of the family on arbitrary datasets.

On the other hand, this ability to separate out subsets of a given dataset is not necessarily driven by the wiggliness or extreme variability of the functions in the family used to model the data. That is, deploying a large collection of rectangles in the plane can separate many (all? see below) subsets of points. Of course, this may not be very practical if the number required grows too fast as the number of points increases, or if given a set of points, it is too hard to readily position the required rectangles.

An obvious generalization here for higher dimensions, using planes and dividing space into little boxes, is exactly the method of decision trees and is thus also a sound approach. The VC dimension of any member of a family of prediction schemes (all decision trees, say) relates to the set of lines or planes being constructed by the method (the tree), and is not a comment about the statistical efficiency (whatever that might mean) of any single line or plane as a decision rule.

Constraining the family to any single line in the plane, on the other hand, shows that the "family" cannot separate out *every* subset of four points arranged as the four points of a square. Constraining the family to all circles in the plane also can't pull out every subset of these four points, but a family of ovals (ellipses) can do so; convince yourself by drawing some squares and ovals surrounding some of the four points.

In fact, to answer this same question for rectangles that we raised above, it can be shown that in the plane *no* set of five points can be separated (shattered) by rectangles; see DGL (chapter 13). Indeed, the VC dimension of rectangles in d-dimensional space is exactly $2d$. More precisely, in the (two-dimensional) plane there are *some* sets of $(2 \times 2 =)$ four points that can be shattered by rectangles, but *no* set of five points can be shattered; see DGL (p. 221).

And while the VC dimension is not known for many possible families of engines, many families do have known VC dimensions, and these known values have very practical consequences. Many such calculations have been done for other classes of machines and these point to a deep combinatorial understanding of model or engine richness or complexity; for details see DGL (chapter 13) and more recently Devroye and Lugosi (2001, chapter 4).

Knowing the VC dimension of a family of models (a class of prediction machines) can allow us to get very specific about tuning the machines. Consider one important example, neural nets having a single hidden layer, and using a threshold sigmoid transfer funcion (see Chapter 3). Given the true VC dimension of this family – sometimes a somewhat complicated function – it is known that the number of hidden inputs should increase as the square root of the sample size. This is specific, practical tuning guidance, and is typical of the amazing power of knowing, even approximately, the VC dimension of a class of machines.

At the other extreme, many families have VC dimension equal to infiinity: given some finite collection of data points in any dimension they can cleanly separate *any* sorting (labeling) of the points into two subsets. For such families the error on a given (training) dataset can be driven down to zero but we will also see the error explode on new (test) data. With such extremely rich families, such as neural nets, we are obligated to moderate – and monitor – the growth of layers and nodes. Since we know the VC dimension of a neural net with any given *finite* set of hidden nodes, this finite number tells us how to grow the network as data is collected.

Sticking with the practical implications of knowing or estimating model richness, it can be shown that using a family with double the VC dimension of another family requires double the sample size of the dataset in order to obtain the same level of predictive accuracy (as precisely quantified in DGL, chapters 12 and 13). This might seem against reason, but the problem here is that a richer family is a bigger family, in effect, a family with more parameters, so more data is required to select the optimal member of the family, or, equivalently, estimate the parameters in the model. On the other hand, keeping the VC dimension fixed but asking to double the accuracy requires getting four times the amount of data. But this result may seem more familiar to data analysts: accuracy goes as the reciprocal of the variance, which itself tracks as the square of the sample size.

2.8 Membership or probability of membership?

Having discussed some of the most general internal aspects of any learning machine, such as its complexity, we turn to the other end of the subject. Namely, what it is that a learning machine is expected to do. Often the biomedical problem of most interest is not the one that first comes to mind. For example, we might start with a pure classification problem {tumor, no tumor} and soon realize that the problem of greatest interest to the patient is not group status precisely, but this query raised by a breast cancer patient: "I understand that I will probably survive five years, but is my chance of surviving 58% or is it closer to 85%?"

This alternative problem is that of estimating the *probability* of belonging to a group (given the data) and is something quite beyond simple group assignment. Some learning machines can, in principle, be reorganized for solving exactly this much harder problem, and still other machines can in retrospect be seen as solving this latter problem even though they were designed for solving the former problem, that of binary prediction.

As a starting point, the very classical machine logistic regression (see Chapter 5 for full details) can be used for *either* the pure classification problem {tumor, no tumor} *or* for estimating the probability of group membership. That is, it can be so used *if* the model specifying the links between features and probability is at least approximately accurate.

On the other hand, Random Forests is an ensemble-learning machine, since it makes predictions by taking a certain majority vote across many predictions. But can *any* such ensemble machine be reconfigured as a provably good probability machine? Can't the actual voting proportion be used as an estimate of the probability of group membership? This is an active area of research; the jury is still out.

Also important to note is the frequent success of the naïve Bayes machine (discussed in Chapter 3). It is clearly based on a probability model, so it might generate good estimates of group membership. In fact, this machine has been an object of study in itself, since the strong assumption of statistical independence among all the features seems so unrealistic; see Zhang (2004). It turns out that this machine's success is evidently due to this phenomenon: we may not need to quite so accurately estimate the true probability of a subject belonging to one group (the control group, say) or the other (the tumor group, say), as long as the inaccurate estimate, the prediction, is *in the right direction*.

Let's see what this means. To better uncover the connection between predicting group status and estimating the probability of group membership, suppose that we decide to put subject y_i in the normal or disease group on the basis of which has the higher estimated probability for group membership. Now, *if* the true probabilities of group membership, given the data, are such that

$$\Pr(\text{disease - free} \mid \text{given the data}) > \Pr(\text{disease} \mid \text{given the data})$$

and *if* our estimate probability from the model is such that

$$\text{estimated } \Pr(\text{disease - free} \mid \text{given the data})$$
$$> \text{true } \Pr(\text{disease - free} \mid \text{given the data})$$

then our decision for group classification will be correct, *even if the estimated probability is far from correct*. Overestimation, in the right direction, comes at no cost in the pure classification problem. Similarly, for classifying a subject as disease group: if we underestimate the probability of group membership, returning a value much less than 0.50, still no error will be made for that subject.

More generally, as long as our estimate of group membership is *anywhere* on the correct side of the decision boundary, a correct decision will still be made. For this reason, with *any* learning machine applied to the classification or prediction problem, we do not necessarily need sharp, exact knowledge of the boundary separating the groups; see Note 5.

This premise of not needing to have sharp, exact knowledge of the decision boundary can be studied quite rigorously, and the larger idea here is that predicting a binary outcome – a group membership – is almost always easier than estimating a continuous outcome, and this includes the problem of estimating the *probability* of group membership. Summarizing, classification is easier than probabilistic function estimation, and is easier also than doing regression (continuous outcome) function estimation; see DGL (section 6.7) for complete details. A basic, somewhat dispiriting finding from deep technical research is that seeking a provably good estimate of the probability of group membership – the Bayes posterior probability – is often too difficult a target in the absence of additional qualifying assumptions about the data.

There is another aspect to this problem of estimating probabilities. It is rather mathematical, but the message is important for practical data analysis. That is, some learning machines that are devised to make good binary {0, 1} decisions have as their technical goal that of minimizing a certain function. These machines can be shown to be excellent decision rules. However, the form of the function deployed could strongly suggest that the machine is, in some provable, deeper sense, a good decision rule *because* it is generating a good estimate of the probability for each subject. For at least one machine, *logitboost*, this suggestion is evidently not valid; see Note 6.

To repeat, keep in mind that a classical logistic regression model (see Chapter 5) will provide probability estimates for each subject, provided the model fits the data. In Section 5.9 we discuss how to interrogate a logistic regression model.

2.9 A taxonomy of machines?

Given the vast and growing sprawl of learning machines – new inventions, sharp improvements on older ones, novel combinations of very different machines – it might be good to have a *taxonomy* of learning machines, a guide to choosing the most appropriate method when dealing with a particular dataset and with a specific goal in mind. Yet the effectiveness of any taxonomy can be questioned. Many of the possible divisions and strata among machines yield taxonomies that only add to the confusion or are irrelevant for a biomedical researcher. Several comments are in order:

(1) One scheme for organizing models could be: *parametric* or *nonparametric*. Upon scrutiny, however, it is seen that some care is required in making this separation precise; see DGL (chapter 16). Another organizing division of species could be *linear* or *nonlinear* models, but this is also surprisingly hard to make precise. That is, if we use methods that are linear combinations of the original features, then a model with interaction terms – products of the original features – is no longer linear in this sense.

(2) Another concern related to model parameters is this: optimal estimation of some parameter in a model (or in a family of models) is really not the same as optimal decision-making. What does this mean? Specifically, a model might require parameter estimation that is done efficiently in order to work properly, and this is the case for familiar linear or logistic regression. But it can be shown that getting a really good parameter estimate is quite distinct from getting a good decision rule if not much is known about the data. That is, the parameter estimate could be satisfyingly close to its true value, but still lead to a not-so-good decision; see DGL (chapter 16).

(3) A further concern related to model parameters is that parameter estimation is good and purposeful when the true model for the data is in the class of data distributions that is being parameterized, or is at least close to it. Expressed another way, if the optimal decision rule is not in the family of all decision rules being studied (whether parametrically or nonparametrically), then the selected (optimally estimated) decision rule can be quite in error. Rather straightforward, simple examples make these arguments quite convincingly; for this also see DGL (chapter 16).

As another way to probe the question of taxonomy, one can pool both neural networks and evolutionary or genetic computing into a class of "biologically" motivated methods, yet this classification doesn't really work either, for several reasons:

(1) First, a stated biological motivation for a single method or approach may not be relevant for solving any given problem. We distinguish here between the biological science of a problem and the choice of a learning machine based on some over-arching biological principle of Nature (granting that such might exist). An analogy applies: the peregrine falcon and the Airbus A380 both fly using wings, but one soars by flapping her wings and the other probably shouldn't. There is, of course, a common element in how both manage to fly – the Bernoulli principle – but the falcon does quite well without such direct knowledge. A flying device or learning machine called *Wings Over Data*, say, may or may not identify the Bernoulli principle and may or may not be relevant for non-airborne problems. The point, finally, is that nonzero skepticism is always required in the presence of lively promotion of a biological narrative to advance one statistical learning machine or another.

(2) At a mathematical level, neural nets and evolutionary computing, for example, are seemingly distinct methods. Yet many of the simpler neural network models, like Hopfield neural nets, are mathematically equivalent to some of the known optimization methods such as simulated annealing, or, so-called Boltzmann learning machines. Moreover, a neural network can be made sufficiently elaborate and complex to envelope a large fraction of other methods under their sponsorship, for example, kernel methods that can be understood as being contained in some of the neural net models; see DGL (section 30.10). Also, any single decision tree can be expressed as a two-hidden-layer neural net; see DGL (p. 542). Summarizing, we can say that many good machines share DNA.

Therefore, to review, attempts to create a clear taxonomy of learning machines as a data analytic guideline are not very fruitful, and we should take a more practical approach: provide a short description of some of the most commonly used machine learning methods (as above) and examine how they operate when applied to a variety of datasets. Indeed, it is often better to apply a library of methods whenever time and resources allow, rather than to assume we can precisely "know" which one to use. More on how to combine methods and approaches into provably better schemes is given in Chapter 11.

2.10 A note of caution – one of many

Before discussing, in Chapter 3, the gears and levers of several learning machines, and turning the reader loose with one shiny, new device after another (zero to 100 kph in *how* many seconds?), we issue a caution. In the absence of a formal parametric model (e.g., a linear regression with a slope and an intercept), and without the usual security net of verifiable distributional assumptions (e.g., the features and the outcome have a joint bivariate normal distribution), at least half of our brainpower and computing time should be spent in honest and intensive evaluation of the prediction engine working on each dataset. This topic is covered in detail in Chapter 11. A similar warning about the importance of validation and error estimation is routinely posted for conventional parametric models (regression, analysis of variance), but this validation process is even more important given the highly nonlinear, nonparametric setting of most statistical learning machines.

2.11 Highlights from the theory

Despite the dark warnings above, there is a body of technical results informing us about the robust excellence of many learning machines. More precisely, many of these often massively nonparametric methods arrive well-anchored to probability arguments, and good estimates of their accuracy. In fact, there is a large mathematical corpus discussing and evaluating the strengths and weaknesses of one method or another using fully rigorous, marvelously inventive probabilistic and statistical reasoning. This literature seems to be still rather separated from mainstream statistical research, but we believe learning – at least about this literature and its merits – is occurring in applied statistics.

We see that elements of this literature, often very insightful, are both alternatively optimistic and discouraging. These results can help us discard methods that might be technically similar to good ones, but are provably themselves not so good. But, as is often the case using very classical statistical methods, the theory in general can usually only tell us how any method might do as we collect increasingly large amounts of data, and then apply a particular prediction engine to the data. So, the results from theory are often upper bounds on error estimates as the dataset size increases, telling us about how far off we might be, not how close we truly are. Understanding and estimating either kind of error – how close we might be to the lowest possible error for any machine, how far away we might be compared to the best machine for that dataset – is the significant sweat equity requirement for any user of statistical learning machines.

Yet another conclusion derived from the already huge technical literature on machine learning methods is this: classical methods can be quite good if all their underlying assumptions are met, and can be arbitrarily bad when even small departures from the assumptions arise. As just one example, see the discussion of the *linear discriminant* method in Chapter 3. Thus, we can state that learning machines are, broadly speaking, more tolerant of departures from a strict set of largely unverifiable assumptions. There is a standard trade-off operating here: if some precise set of assumptions is known to be, or is plausibly valid for the data, then a sharper inference and more accuracy in prediction is obtained. If the road ahead is known to be fully paved and well marked, then an Audi R8 might be a good choice; otherwise a pack mule or camel or dog sled is suggested.

Let's see what else is known from the theoretical studies. These findings do not answer directly the *Twenty Canonical Questions* given in Chapter 1. They are, instead, directed at the reader interested in seeing what theory has been able to derive that can help us in *entirely practical ways*. They are given here to promote the study of the subject itself for the more technically well-prepared, or at least the fearless, and to display the stunning advances in the field that may not be so widely known.

Below, certain technical terms remain not perfectly defined, for example *Bayes consistency*. For now just think of this important property as the lowest possible prediction error if given all possible information about the data.

Let's begin.

(1) Many good machine methods exist, but if the one with very low prediction error requires enormous amounts of data, you might get very close to a perfectly good result with a smaller, more cost-effective machine. This is the issue of the *rate of convergence*, or, how effectively a given machine makes use of data. For any verifiably good method (that

is, a Bayes consistent method, with lowest possible prediction error), there are configurations of data (distributions) that require arbitrarily large amounts of data in order to be close to the optimal, lowest error value that the machine provides; DGL (chapter 6) covers this topic.

(2) Benchmarking, in the limited sense of using real or simulated data to compare the absolute performance of any two machines, is probably a waste of time. Theory discussed in DGL (chapter 7) has this to report: suppose we are given Machine A, some number n, and any small positive number c, with $\frac{1}{2} > c > 0$. Then there exists data with sample size n drawn from some distribution, such that the error probability for Machine A is at least $\frac{1}{2} - c$. This result is foundational in the literature, so let's take it apart:

   (a) the result asks for no information whatsover about the workings of Machine A;

   (b) the Bayes risk for the distribution is, by construction in this example, exactly zero;

   (c) we may use *any* distribution with Bayes risk zero for this result;

   (d) the result holds for any chosen sample size n;

   (e) the conclusion is that the Bayes risk for Machine A is stuck arbitrarily close to $\frac{1}{2}$, that is, marginally only slightly better than random coin tossing, on that dataset.

(3) Here is another version of the dilemma posed by (2). Again, suppose we are given any Machine A. Then there always exist another Machine B, and a distribution such that the probability of error for Machine B is always strictly less than that for Machine A, for every sample size. Let's also take this apart:

   (a) once again nothing is assumed about the inner workings of Machine A;

   (b) the better Machine B is shown to be strongly Bayes consistent – given enough data, from *any* distribution, the probability of error for Machine B can be driven arbitrarily close to the minimum possible error for that distribution, that is the Bayes error (which may in fact not be zero);

   (c) as in (2) above the result holds for data with any sample size.

(4) Combining (2) and (3) we find: there are provably no super classifiers, no universally superior classifiers. The continuing, sprawling literature verifying that today's Quite Clever Machine is *uniformly* better than any

Shabby Machine from Yesterday, because *this* dataset tells us so, is largely a waste of time and brainpower.

(5) On the other hand, there do exist machine families that are strongly uniformly Bayes consistent, in the sense that given enough data from any distribution the error can be driven to the Bayes minimum (for the data), and this occurs no matter what the structure or other properties of the data happen to be. We state machine families here since we need to tune the engine as data is collected, and this tuning shifts us from one member of the family to another in a carefully graduated way. Also, careful inspection here reveals that this result doesn't contradict the result described in (2) or (3), since those arguments specifically require the distribution and dataset to be modified as the constants n and c are changed.

(6) So, instead of the pointless search for the optimal machine for all data, or the nearly equally fruitless search for finding the very best machine (from among some usually highly select, small collection) for a given dataset, we see that studying machines on different data can help us understand how an individual machine works as it does, what it responds to best in the data, and what it doesn't properly account for in the data; see Chapter 4. One instance of this: an *SVM* (= support vector machine; see Chapter 3) doesn't see – is insensitive to – data far outside the *margin*, away from a zone near the true decision boundary, that line or surface approximately separating the two groups. Is this a good thing? It also doesn't see the group means. Is that what we want? Sometimes yes, sometimes no.

(7) Finding good parameter estimates for optimizing a machine (or statistical model, like linear regression) is not at all the same as finding the best machine. In other words, minimum parameter error is not the same as minimum probability of error, or even minimum error in estimating the probability of group membership. Here is the context for this distinction: the parameter estimates required to define and then run the machine could be, for example, the coefficients in a logistic regression model. And the probability of error in prediction is the percentage of incorrectly classified subjects, while the probability of group membership is our estimate of the chance that the subject belongs to one group or the other. Continuing with this idea ...

(8) Minimum error probability is not the same as minimum error in estimation of probability of group membership. Translating into plain text: we can be seriously wrong about estimating the correct probability of group membership (you don't have a 58% chance of survival over five years, as the machine predicts, but actually an 85% chance) and still have perfect (zero error) scores in decision-making (in pure classification terms: you are predicted to most likely survive and this is highly accurate). So, when does one imply the other? This is a fundamental area of current research, see Note 6.

(9) Many *very* primitive machines often, provably, do very well and require exactly no parameter estimation at all. Thus, the *cubic histogram*, *statistically balanced blocks* – for which see DGL (chapters 9 and 21) – and *nearest neighbors*, all do very well, in that each has no data-dependent parameters for running on a given dataset.

(10) Some primitive but excellent methods often still need some user modifications as the data sample size, N, increases. The reason is that as N gets large the local nature of the method needs to be adjusted, but not too fast: this adjustment must be done at proper pace. Thus, a delicate balance in this dance to infinity is required to get provably best results. Further translation of this result: most machines need to be increasingly local as data is collected in order to make the most informed vote. The rate at which they must burrow into the data is usually a function of the amount of data available and the local peculiarities of the data. But even knowing nothing about the data in advance, many machines are good when enough data is collected, though their accuracy can be sharpened by the dance. Here's an example: for the k-nearest-neighbor method (see Chapter 3), the value k needs to get larger as N does, but carefully, so that the ratio k/N has to go to zero as N gets large. Note that this adjustment in the choice of number of neighbors is *not* data-dependent, and only sample-size-dependent: no parameter has to be estimated using any other aspects of the data itself.

(11) A prediction machine that is probably not good (is not provably Bayes consistent) can still generate a provably good machine when it is used as a basic part of a committee machine (*Random Forests* and *Random Jungles* are like this), or when it is melded into a sequential scheme such as *boosting*. The base classifiers in boosting, for example, are often

elemental trees with a single split (so, in isolation, are usually not optimal), but the tiny trees are assigned weights as the scheme is iterated. In fact, these weights are modified as the iteration moves forward, and the data itself is progressively reweighted. Despite being premised on tiny trees, this complex system of weights is known to be Bayes consistent; see Lugosi and Vayatis (2004).

Moreover, some forms of Random Forests are *not* provably Bayes consistent. The reason here is that if the individual trees use the method of *splitting to purity* then the terminal nodes at the bottom of the trees end up with too few observations. With too few observations surrounding a new data point, getting a good prediction of group membership is that much harder. Parallel to this, the elementary, base classifier in a boosting scheme may be a "tree" with a single split, a so-called stump, which in itself is deeply primitive and generally not Bayes consistent.

Yet again, some small adjustments to these schemes, to Random Forests for example, may result in provable Bayes consistency. The twin morals here: tiny changes can recast a weak method as a good one, and averaging over many imperfect rules (such as over a collection of single, stumpy decision trees) can do this as well.

(12) Finally, we can report from the theory that *any* consistent machine (one having the best possible error values as more data is collected) is necessarily local, and is always good in a very weak global sense; see Zakai and Ritov, 2008, 2009. Let's sort this out:

(a) Consistent here means what it does above – given data from any distribution the machine gets arbitrarily close to the Bayes error value as more data is collected.

(b) The idea of information being basically local here is sensible but also requires some modification as more data is collected. That is, local means a small neighborhood around the test point at which prediction or estimation is required. The neighborhood includes some small portion of the original data, and the size of the neighborhood is assumed to get smaller as more data is collected. This is another version of the dance to infinity.

(c) That any Bayes consistent method must necessarily be local is from a biomedical data point of view, unremarkable. How a test point should be classified often depends on the surrounding points in the data and should not be affected very much by points that are far away. But from a technical perspective this result is *very* surprising, since important prediction engines – support vector machines and boosting, for example – do not have any obvious locality built into their mathematical definition. So, the deeper point is that good machines should do nearly as well when given only a local neighborhood of the test point.

(d) The weak global condition that is also a property of any consistent scheme is that it should estimate the overall mean value of all the *outcomes* in the data. Given data of the form $\{y, x\}$ for lots of ys and xs, where we want to use the xs to predict or estimate the ys, a necessary (but certainly not sufficient) property of the consistent machine is that it only has to predict the mean value of the ys sufficiently accurately. In fact, a not-good machine can always be arranged to satisfy this property: just ignore all the xs and take the sample mean of the ys. In the setting where we want the machine to make good estimates of y, given x (the regression setting), such a silly machine does do this task. And a similar, but equally silly prediction machine can be devised as well. Both of these machines satisfy the weak global property but surely not the locality property we described above as they don't even *see* any of the xs.

(e) And here is the summary of this amazing local/global result from the theory: given good local behavior and the weak global property on the data, these are enough to prove consistency for all data. But mind the important footnote: we've only loosely sketched a notion of localizable above, and considerable precision is required to show the equivalence of consistency with certain local and global properties. It can be shown, for example, that there exists a machine that is consistent but is neither localizable nor locally consistent; see Zakai and Ritov (2009), Proposition 1. Do not expect such technical statements as these to be quickly assimilated; there is real and deep art flowing through these methods.

Notes

(1) A continuous outcome produced (generated, calculated) by a learning machine can also be this: an estimated value for the probability of

belonging to a group. In this situation we might use a learning machine to state that this patient has, for example, an 85% probability of having a cancerous colon polyp. As discussed in several places in this text, these two activities, declaring membership or estimating probability of membership, are not equivalent.

(2) A final note on terminology: in our experience any research paper having in its title any of the words, *unique, flexible, general, powerful, revolutionary*, is often none of these.

(3) Of course, if statistical or other structural assumptions about the data can be invoked then often more precise inferences (decisions) can be made. This is the typical trade-off between prior information about data structure and the power of the ultimate inference or conclusion. Here, a Bayesian argument would insist that all this initial information be expressed in probability terms; see for example Gelman *et al.* (2004). A less programmatic description of this process is that some balanced combination of more data or stricter assumptions about the data is required to make good decisions. If we don't have much data then we need to make more assumptions, and bring in more subject-matter information to proceed.

Less comprehensively, linear regression and discriminant analysis are classical examples of parametric prediction engines, where the parameter list is usually quite small, and we often assume that the data has a multivariate normal distribution. As expected, the starting assumptions then lead to refined inference about the individual parameters in these models. Except for the Bayesian machines described in Chapter 3, and these classical linear models, we do not in this text make distributional assumptions, either prior to data collection, or after inspection of the data. Too often, in our experience, simply trying to validate the set of entangled, underlying assumptions being posited is a low-power, ineffective procedure.

(4) Unsupervised learning is discussed in many places, including Hastie *et al.* (2009); see also the recent, and very detailed study by Getoor and Taskar (2007). There is an expanding literature on the important problems of comparing clusters, and evaluating the overlap of networks or biological pathways; see, for example, Forti and Foresti (2006), Minku and Ludermir (2008). We strongly encourage the mathematically fearless to help develop this area, bringing some measure of statistical validation to the project.

(5) Let's make this more precise. Suppose as given, the problem of classifying into one of two groups, A or B. Given the data, x, let the *true* probability of belonging to A be written as $n(x)$, so

$n(x) = \text{Pr(subject belongs to Group } A, \text{given the data } x).$

Then by the usual probability rule,

$1 - n(x) = \text{Pr(subject belongs to Group } B, \text{given the data } x).$

Good estimation of this unknown group membership function $n(x)$ is then the target of statistical learning machines for the classifcation problem. That is, if $n(x)$ were known exactly, and if we decided that the ith subject is a member of Group A only whenever $n(x) > \frac{1}{2}$, then we would have a *Bayes optimal decision rule*. Here optimal means that given any *other* decision rule $g(x)$ that tries to estimate the probability of group membership (is my chance of survival 58% or 85%?), it can be demonstrated that

$\text{Pr(subject is misclassified using rule } g(x))$
$\geq \text{Pr(subject is misclassified using rule } n(x)).$

In words, the probability of misclassification using anything other than the true membership function must go up. However, if we choose to not attempt estimating the membership function, and only make a pure decision given the data, the problem changes, and generally is much easier. For this problem we only need a function of the data such that $g(x) = 1$, say, when we declare the subject to be in Group A, and:

$g(x) = 1$ whenever $n(x) > \frac{1}{2}$,
$g(x) = 0$ whenever $n(x) < \frac{1}{2}$,
$g(x) = $ randomly 1 or 0 whenever $n(x) = \frac{1}{2}$.

In words, our rule $g(x)$ only needs to be on the correct *side* of the decision boundary, and then randomly equal to 1 or 0 when $n(x) = \frac{1}{2}$.

(6) The two recent studies of Mease *et al.* (2007, 2008) are essential reading for this problem, which gets technical rather quickly, so we summarize the main issues.

It is observed that the quite-good learning machine *logitboost* is defined by its effort to minimize a certain exponential function, as it proceeds iteratively; see Section 3.8 for more on boosting generally. And the true minimum of this (loss) function, when taken over all possible real-valued functions, is indeed directly convertible to the probability of group membership. However, several elementary examples provided by Mease *et al.* also show that logitboost evidently does not do a good job of estimating the probabilities themselves directly. What is going on here?

One perspective on the problem is that logitboost, as a learning machine, when constructed by minimizing the functional, is doing a search in a much smaller space of functions than the whole space of real-valued functions that are bounded by 0 and 1. This vastly bigger space includes the (conditional) probability function we're trying to estimate. Which is to say that the logitboost minimum may or may not be close to the true, unconstrained minimum, which we know lives somewhere out there in the big space. Indeed, logitboost can be seen (Devroye, personal communication) as a type of neural network – a multilayer perceptron – with one hidden layer; see DGL (chapter 30) for the precise details about this family of machines.

But the complexity of all such neural networks, as measured by the VC dimension for this family, has an upper and lower bound (both probably sharp) determined by the number of nodes in the hidden layer and the dimension of the problem, that is, the number of features. And it is futher known that in order to do well, using *any* scheme for estimating the machine's parameters (the weights in the sum over all the two-node trees that appear in logitboost), the sample size must be much larger than the VC dimension; see DGL (section 30.4). Summarizing, logitboost is probably not complex enough – by itself – to be certain to estimate the true real-valued function that minimizes the exponential function. It *might* close to the minimum, for *some* datasets, but theory developed to date does not support the premise that it does so uniformly for all data, or for realistic sample sizes. That is, it *might* generate a good estimate of the group membership probability for each subject, but theory currently suggests it's certainly not guaranteed to do so.

And the simple examples of Mease *et al.* (2007, 2008) (as well as several of our own, not shown here) all point in the wrong direction: logitboost seems to work – and indeed it does work very well as a pure binary decision rule – by pushing the estimated probabilities for each subject toward the two extremes, 0 and 1. It thus functions as an excellent binary rule, but not so good as a probability machine. In fact, doing well at the first problem seems to preclude doing very well at the second problem, or at least it is not so implied; see the discussion in Note 5 above.

It is only fair to note that pushing estimated probabilities around as part of making good binary decisions is not limited to logitboost. Simple simulations (not shown) reveal that Random Forests also has this property, though perhaps not so strikingly.

There is tantalizing theory already available – at least for the mathematically fearless – suggesting that some forms of post-processing for logitboost, or Random Forests, might ultimately get us to good probability estimates. See DGL, section 30.8, where neural nets are shown to be expandable (by adding one or two more layers of hidden nodes) to schemes that are certain to be good estimators of any bounded real function. Here, as at many other places, monitoring the VC dimension of the proposed scheme is critical *and* fairly sharp bounds are already known for the VC dimension for these schemes. In fact, the theory points to results for many other schemes, apart from logitboost, at least suggesting that they could be post-processed into being good probability estimators. Clearly, more work remains to be done here.

Evidently the only practical machine for the second problem, that of probability estimation, is something akin to the classical logistic regression model, if the model is at least close to being correct in the first place. So, finally, doing well in this probability estimation context means two things: (a) finding a relatively small set of features to use as input and then (b) generating the goodness-of-fit measures, as studied by Kuss (2002) and Hu et al. (2006), in order to validate the original assumption that we have something close to the correct model; for more on this validation process see Chapter 5.

3

A mangle of machines

Avoid strange and unfamiliar words as a sailor avoids rocks at sea.
From *On Analogy*, by Julius Caesar (ca. 54 BCE)

Barring that natural expression of villainy which we all have, the machine looked honest enough.
(With apologies to Mark Twain)

3.1 Introduction

Our survey covers learning machines that have been studied intensively and applied widely. We do not focus on detailed discussion of the numerous versions of each, and we barely cover the full spectrum of learning machines now available; see Note 1. The goal of this chapter is to display the set of core ideas that propel each method. We also do not linger over the mathematical details and, as before, we make an effort to sharply limit any viewing of the mathematical details; see Note 2.

3.2 Linear regression

A simple classification or prediction method can often be obtained by fitting a linear regression model. It is a very classical and still very important method.

Let the *outcome* be y and the single *predictor* be x. Then *linear regression* of y on x is written as:

$$y = a + bx,$$

where the constants a and b have to be estimated from the data. The next step up in generality is to allow for multiple predictors:

$$x_1, x_2, \ldots, x_k,$$

where the x_i can be any collection of discrete or continuous predictors. In this case the prediction equation has the form:

$$y = a + b_1 x_1 + b_2 x_2 + \ldots + b_k x_k,$$

for constants $a, b_1, b_2, \ldots, b_k$. This collection of constants forms the parameters of this linear model – they are estimated from the data, and one method for doing so is that of least squares. Here, the constants are selected such that the difference between the observed y and the estimated y (denoted $\hat{y}$) is minimized using a sum of squares criterion; see for example Berk (2008), which discusses regression in the context of learning machines. The result takes the form:

$$\hat{y} = \hat{a} + \hat{b}_1 x_1 + \hat{b}_2 x_2 + \ldots + \hat{b}_k x_k,$$

for estimates $\hat{a}, \hat{b}_1, \hat{b}_2, \ldots \hat{b}_k$.

It is remarkable that a simple additive and linear model like this can be so broadly effective in real-world data analysis. Indeed, there is a body of critical thinking in the statistical community asserting that linear, additive models, using small sets of predictors, can do nearly as well as many recently developed statistical learning machines – but see Note 3.

This basic least-squares approach assumes very little about the data – apart from the assumption of being linear in the data, which itself may be nontrivial. For sufficiently large amounts of data the method is known to be statistically optimal (in a precise sense that we don't engage here), and estimates of the model parameters are approximately normally distributed. If additional distributional properties of the data are assumed – such as that the $(y, x_1, x_2, \ldots, x_k)$ are multivariate normal – then classical statistical inference can be applied to generate statistical statements about the parameters, for any size dataset. Finally then, confidence intervals and classical hypothesis tests for the parameters can be generated.

Linear regression is simple, easy to implement, widely available, but is somewhat sensitive to outliers and is unlikely to accommodate complicated decision boundaries; see Chapter 7.

3.3 Logistic regression

A method closely related to linear regression is *logistic regression*. It is a foundational method in the analysis of biological data, and we discuss it in detail in its own chapter: Chapter 5. In the basic version of this model the outcome y is binary $\{0, 1\}$ and designates a subject's group membership, the status of the patient, the status of a cell sample {tumor, not tumor}. Logistic regression can also be extended to multiple group outcomes. The model can equivalently be expressed as a method for predicting the probability of group membership, that is, the model generates an estimate of the probability that the patient belongs to one of the two groups: this patient has an estimated 85% chance of belonging to the non-tumor group. Then, after a transformation, this probability of group membership can be written as a linear model. This is a very important idea.

Indeed, this distinction between group prediction (belongs to the tumor group, belongs to the non-tumor group) and the estimation of group membership probability is strictly nontrivial. However, the transformation between the two under logistic regression is seamless, under the strict premise that the model – these features combined in this way – is the true model; see Section 2.7.

For the classification engines we discuss in this book, logistic regression is the default "simple" model for predicting a subject's group status. As discussed in Chapter 12, it can be applied after a more complex learning machine has done the heavy lifting of identifying an important small set of predictors given a very large list of candidate predictors. It could also be included as a "measurement" in a learning machine, so that predictions from one machine can be folded into the input for other machines. *Calibrating* a logistic regression invokes this approach, by folding the result of one logistic regression into another; see Section 5.9.

3.4 Linear discriminant

Though not often presented as such, this very classical method can be viewed as a form of linear regression, such that a collection of features

$$x = (x_1, x_2, \ldots, x_k)$$

is used to predict a binary outcome $y = 0$, or 1. The *discriminant function* has the form:

$$y = w_0 + w_1 x_1 + w_2 x_2 + \ldots + w_k x_k,$$

where $w = (w_0, w_1, w_2, \ldots, w_k)$ is a collection of parameters to be estimated. The discriminant function is then a single number, such that if greater than zero, subject assignment is made to one group, and if less than or equal to zero, assignment is made to the other group. The method by which the function is calculated takes into account the correlation structure of the measurements $x = (x_1, x_2, \ldots, x_k)$. That is, the correlations between the components, the features, x_i and x_j for all i and j, are estimated (or specified by the user) and then incorporated into the estimation of the model coefficients. If the correlation structures in the two groups are thought to be different, then a *quadratic discriminant* function can be applied instead; see Kendall 1980.

This scheme provably yields the best discrimination (sharpest group separation) when the data consist of two Gaussian (normally distributed) groups. Its purpose is to locate that line or plane that best separates the two groups. There are similarities here with linear support vector machines; see Figure 3.1.

As with regression methods generally, it can also be very sensitive to outliers; see Chapter 8. More recently, methods have been developed that combine the linear discriminant with so-called kernel methods, and yield robust kernel linear discriminants. These serve to model the data in a relatively simple, linear form and also minimize the consequences of discordant observations.

Small departures from the assumptions (of two normally distributed groups) could be remedied using more robust methods as just described, but another working assumption is often that *some* other linear model could still be found to nicely separate the groups, and that perhaps the linear model approach (to finding the coefficients in the linear equation for the model) would not be far from this alternative model. This is utterly mistaken and exactly correct, depending on what is meant by *linear*.

That is, it is provably the case that there are "linear models" such that given enough data they can drive the Bayes error to zero. Notably, *linear* in this case means a collection of *functions of the data* combined in a linear fashion; these are so-called generalized additive models, see DGL (chapter 17).

Yet it is also true for some specific datasets that the standard linear discriminant model has an error that is arbitrarily close to one, and is then nearly twice as bad as random coin-tossing. Indeed, in this case, the data *is* fully separated by some linear equation (a hyperplane) just not a classical discriminant equation; see DGL (problem 4.9).

3.5 Bayes classifiers – regular and naïve

A Bayes classifier is a probabilistic learning scheme that begins with a choice of priors. Priors are probabilities for group membership before data is collected, and often, more grandly, also probabilities for different models or states of Nature. Then an argument from classical probability generates the conditional probability of observing a particular outcome *given* the predictors and the priors. (This is a mouthful – bear with us.)

These probabilistic values – the priors – can be estimated from a preliminary or provisional data. However, even given these priors directly, the full-strength Bayes classifier then requires a second step, calculating the posterior probabilities for group membership, given the data and the priors. This critical second step is technically nontrivial and computationally demanding, and has historically thwarted the broad application of Bayes methods to datasets of any significant size. The purely computational issues have eased dramatically in the last two decades due to dramatic increases in computing power. However, we still often see that a Bayes classifier requires larger amounts of data than other methods to achieve the same level of model accuracy. Put simply, this difficulty can be understood as the combined challenge of the several steps: estimating prior probabilities, and then conducting a multidimensional integration problem (recall your calculus class, where necessary); see Gelman *et al.* (2004). Carlin and Louis (2000) The general Bayes approach is fundamentally, philosophically different from the so-called frequentist method, so that model fitness and error comparison with other procedures can be difficult to make; for more on this distinction between statistical approaches, see Berger and Wolpert (1988), Pace and Salvan (1997), Welsh (1996).

Bayes methods have an enormous literature, a long and storied history, and a still-advancing army of vocal adherents. On the other hand, the two approaches (frequentist and Bayes) often lead to basically the same inference, and indeed, there is a school of statistical thinking that suggests any "good" frequentist model should also be derivable under a Bayesian outlook.

Having commented on assumptions, priors, posteriors, calculus problems, and computing overhead, we now direct the reader to a recent variant of the Bayes classifier, the so-called *naïve Bayes* method. It assumes statistical independence of all the features: at a very minimum this means the features are assumed to all be uncorrelated with each other. In particular, any biological interactions among the features (genes, alleles, single nucleotide polymorphisms, clinical data) are set to zero. This is often a wildly implausible assumption, but the method has been shown to work surprisingly well; see, for example, Zhang (2004b).

To proceed further into our description of the naïve Bayes approach, we need to get more technical. That is, the method constrains the probability of observing a particular outcome given a set of predictors to be just a simple *product* of the probabilities conditioned on individual predictors. More formally, suppose we want to predict the probability of an outcome y given a collection of predictors $\{x_1, x_2, \ldots, x_k\}$. Then the prediction is:

$$\Pr(y \mid x_1, x_2, \ldots, x_k) = C \times \Pr(y) \times \Pr(x_1 \mid y) \times \Pr(x_2 \mid y) \times \ldots \\ \times \Pr(x_k \mid y).$$

The constant C here is the reciprocal of the probability of the set of predictors taking on the values $\{x_1, x_2, \ldots, x_k\}$. And each term in the product is a conditional probability, but is reversed: they are estimates of the probability of the predictor having value x, given y. For example, the probability of a SNP having value $\{1\}$ and not $\{0\}$, given that the tissue has status $\{tumor\}$. Each of the conditional probabilities $\Pr(x_i \mid y)$ is estimated from the data and the product yields the estimated probability for y. Of course, a fully Bayesian analysis usually does not impose the constraint of functional independence for each of the conditional probabilities. In the general situation the full dependence (or at least correlation) structure of the features needs to be part of the model assumptions or well estimated from the data.

A warning: in order to make this method computationally efficient, especially with large numbers of predictors, it is usually assumed that the predictors are themselves discrete, or can be made discrete in some sensible way. In fact, the data typically needs to be just binary, $\{0 \text{ or } 1\}$. Yet, in statistical inference generally, turning a continuous predictor into a discrete or binary one, by dividing up the range of values for that predictor, for example, is well known for leading to inaccurate or at least inefficient estimation. Some numerical experimentation with this *binning* process (placing measurement values into distinct bins, $1 \leq x < 2$, $2 \leq x < 3$, etc.) is warranted if undertaken, as the choice of bin could dramatically affect the ultimate inference and the predictions.

3.6 Logic regression

A recently developed method is *logic regression*; see Ruczinski *et al.* (2003), Kooperberg and Ruczinski (2005).

This terminology might be confusing, as it is a method quite distinct from the more familiar *logistic regression*, discussed in Chapter 5. Indeed, we would like to refer to this method as *Boolean logic regression*, but that only further muddles the landscape, so logic regression it must be.

In this approach a model is developed that relates the predictors to the response, a binary outcome, but actively introduces new predictors. These new predictors can model quite complex interactions between the predictors, but the interactions are typically kept simple (as with standard two or three-way interactions in a fixed effects analysis of variance). Note that theory here doesn't limit the number of possible interactions, but practicality does, and we believe it becomes quite hard to interpret such higher-order models – three-way interactions are hard enough for us. However, if our central, stated goal is that of predicting the outcome, that is the group membership of a subject, then we need not limit ourselves in this primary step in the analysis.

Here's how it works. We start with a set of binary (0, 1) predictors (features) and create new binary predictors by considering all logical (so-called *Boolean*) combinations of the original predictors. Suppose A and B are two of the original predictors (clinical results from two tests, or, values for two SNPs, etc.). Then new predictors P_1, P_2, P_3, can take the form:

$P_1(A, B) = \{A \text{ OR } B\}$ which is 1 if $A = 1$ OR $B = 1$, and is 0 otherwise;

$P_2(A, B) = \{A \text{ AND } B\}$ which is 1 if $A = 1$ AND $B = 1$, and is 0 otherwise;

$P_3(A) = \{NOT\ A\}$ *which is* 1 *if* $A = 0$, and is 0 when $A = 1$.

These three predictors can then in turn be combined (compounded) in quite complex ways to yield new (Boolean logic) features, such as this one:

$$f(A, B, C, D) = \{(A \text{ OR } B) \text{ OR } (\text{NOT } (C \text{ AND } D))\} \text{ OR } (B \text{ AND } C)$$
$$= \{P_1(A, B) \text{ OR } (\text{NOT } P_2(C, D))\} \text{ OR } \{P_2(B, C)\}.$$
$$= P_1[\{P_1(A, B) \text{ OR } P_3(P_2(C, D))\}, P_2(B, C)]$$
$$= P_1[\{P_1\{P_1(A, B), P_3(P_2(C, D))\}, P_2(B, C)\}].$$

The motivating premise is that, as part of a prediction scheme, such new logical binary features might be more adapted to capturing the interactivity of one binary feature with another.

More concretely, we might suspect that SNP1 and SNP2 are involved with genes that are interacting promoters or regulators for generation of a protein related to the underlying disease being studied {tumor, not tumor}. Then a new logical operator could be included as a feature:

$$f(\text{SNP1}, \text{SNP2}) = \{\text{SNP1 AND } (\text{NOT SNP2})\} \text{ OR}$$
$$\{(\text{NOT SNP1}) \text{ AND SNP2}\}$$
$$= P_1[P_2\{\text{SNP1}, P_3(\text{SNP2})\}, P_2\{P_3(\text{SNP1}), \text{SNP2}\}].$$

As we see, these logical operators start to look very complicated, very quickly. The logic regression algorithm is not much troubled by this complexity, so we need not be either. The important idea here is that the user is not specifically required to invent these logical features, as the logic regression program does that on the fly, and in a controlled manner.

It can be shown that any Boolean statement such as $f(A,B)$ can be represented graphically as a *decision tree*; see Chapter 6.

An important aspect of logic regression is that there are no logical or subject-matter restrictions on the complexity of the new logical expressions $f(A,B)$. The process of curtailing the rampant introduction of new logical expressions is program-code-dependent – there isn't a mathematical limit on the introduction but an important computational one. Another question that can't be answered directly by the method is indeed whether or not interactions between any features can always be effectively defined by Boolean logical expressions. We leave this for further research.

3.7 *k*-Nearest neighbors

A generally very good, yet very simple learning machine method is that of *k-nearest neighbors (k-NN)*. It is unashamedly a primitive scheme as it does not require any statistical or probabilistic assumptions and is easy to understand. Yet there is deep technical theory showing that it can perform remarkably well; see DGL (chapters 5 and 11). That such theoretical results can be obtained, with truly no statistical assumptions, is itself an object of wonder; such is the state of the art for *probabilistic pattern recognition.*

The basic idea itself is rather convincing on its own: classification of a subject should depend on the local neighborhood of that subject. Hence, if a data point is surrounded by many "not survive" instances then it too should be classified as "not survive." Now, while this is an excellent idea in principle, it still asks that we define a *neighborhood,* and in turn that means we have to specify a *distance measure* between the individual subjects: recall our earlier discussion of unsupervised learning and similarity, in Sections 2.2, 2.3, and 2.4.

A standard choice is the Euclidean distance, where each predictor is treated as a component in the (possibly high-dimensional) feature space. The *neighborhood* is found by searching the known examples for similar data (case or control, say) and identifying a predefined number, k, of the "closest" neighbors. Voting then occurs over these nearest neighbors, with the majority vote making the decision. Finally, while the assignment of the class is made solely based on the properties of these neighbors, modifications to the assignment can be made using a weighting function, for which the weight of a neighbor is a function of the local distance to that neighbor. Of course, as new data points are added, the neighborhoods will evolve, necessitating new distance calculations and weights. Also important is that the distance function may not be obvious and there already exists an enormous library of such functions, successfully applied in one subject-matter area after another; see Chapter 2. On the other hand, there is research showing that the good choice of the distance function can be based on the data itself: see DGL (chapter 26, theorem 26.3).

The next important question to ask is: given the distance function, how do we make a good selection of k? That is, how "deep" should the local neighborhoods be? Besides being dependent on the data itself, a more general fact is that larger values of k are smoothing the boundary between the classes, since the voting is taking place over a larger neighborhood. This may or may not be a good thing. A good choice for k can be selected by some parameter optimization technique, for example, evolutionary and genetic algorithms or cross-validation; see DGL (chapter 5), for more of the technical details. Deep results from theory provide guidance on how k should be selected, namely, it should increase as the size of the dataset increases, but not too fast.

One alternative version of a neighborhood could involve just defining many subsets of the data, a partition of all the data points. Each new subject then appears in some small box, and this generates a classification for that point. This is the basic idea behind the classification and regression tree approach, of Random Forests, Random Jungles, and other methods: see Chapter 7. Indeed, Random Forests can be identified as a kind of adaptive nearest-neighbor scheme: see DGL (chapter 11, problem 11.6), Lin and Jeon (2006). Again we see that routinely effective learning machines will likely share DNA.

In general, the k-nearest-neighbors algorithm is easy to implement, although computationally intensive, especially when the size of the data grows. This is due to the fact that, for classifying the next subject, it requires the calculation of that subject's distances from all the other cases.

3.8 Support vector machines

Support vector machines (*SVMs*) belong to the large group of so-called *kernel methods*. They have become quite popular and this is likely a result of three factors: (i) the mathematical elegance of the method; (ii) the deep theoretical work of Vapnik, Chervonenkis, and others, showing the statistical optimality of the method under very general conditions; and (iii) the success of the scheme for a very large variety of datasets. We don't discuss most of the inner workings of the mathematics of the method and don't discuss at all the theory leading to the invention of the approach. For this, see DGL (chapter 10), and more recently the work of Steinwart (2005). This paper demonstrates that SVMs, and the entire class of so-called regularized kernel classifiers, are Bayes consistent: with some data-dependent tuning these methods come arbitrarily close to the lowest possible error value as data is collected. This is nontrivial, technical material and instead we discuss the approach using only broad strokes and central themes; for more see Cristianini and Shawe-Taylor (2000), Schölkopf and Smola (2002), along with Schölkopf *et al.* (2001)

A linear support vector machine is displayed in Figure 3.1.

One of the main ideas here is that the original features can be used to systematically and quickly generate new features, and do so in a very organized way. This is especially important if the original features do not suggest a simple linear or plane separation between the groups. Then it might be possible that some transformation of the features could lead to a linear separation, in the transformed data space.

It is possible to introduce a very large family of such new features in a very systematic way, using so-called *kernel functions*. These functions act like new distance measures on the data points. The new functions belong to mathematically related families, such as linear, quadratic, polynomial, or exponential functions. And the functions may be combined in many ways to generate additional kernels. A very important consequence of working with kernel functions is that they can be computed quickly. There is, therefore, a superficial similarity here with the Boolean logic regression approach, as both introduce new features in an organized way, but for SVMs neither the

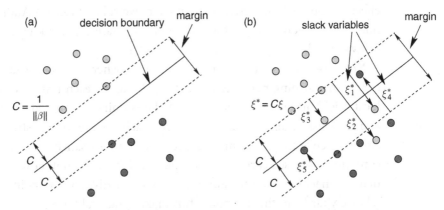

Figure 3.1.   (a) How two groups might be separated using a single decision boundary, in this case a straight line, where the groups are fully separable. The SVM finds that line that maximizes the margin. The parameter C is estimated from the data, and $\|\beta\|$ is the length of the estimated parameter vector in the model. (b) Shows data that is not fully separable using a single line. Here the margin is found by using so-called slack variables, which account for data near to, or on the "wrong" side of the line. This standard case allows for user-input as to the importance of these slack variables in the final model.

original nor the new features need be binary in their outcome, nor require using binary values as inputs.

Another key idea is that perhaps only points near the true decision boundary should really matter; recall that we introduced this idea in our discussion in Section 2.9. These truly critical points are said to be in the *margin* of the support vector rule, for a given kernel function, if they are not too far from the boundary, even if they might be on the "wrong" side. An SVM with a given kernel is then a machine that maximizes this margin, while trying to limit the prediction error in the model. As always there is a trade-off in these twin goals, and the relative proportion of the goals is assigned through a user-input parameter.

Thus, the mathematics of an SVM has an alternative formulation that relates directly to this proposition. Namely, that the coefficients in the model are constrained (smoothed) through a user-specified, often data-dependent parameter. This is the regularization idea, otherwise expressed, and this kind of interconnectivity of the several possible defining equations for an SVM is a source of its technical elegance. We caution the user, here as elsewhere, to keep elegance in perspective: an elegant method may be exactly the least effective approach to a given dataset – a powerful and elegant Audi A5 may not be much good on an otherwise perfectly maintained hiking trail in the Schwarzwald.

Note also our discussion in Section 2.11, where we observed that any consistent learning machine needs to be local: for each test point only the local neighborhood of the data needs to be examined. As noted above, SVMs and the class of all suitably regularized machines are indeed strongly consistent. Hence they, too, must act locally and also satisfy the weak global condition discussed earlier. This property of locality is another way of saying that the machine is robust and relatively insensitive to data points that are relatively far from the test point: this makes practical sense.

Finally, we note that those data points that are exactly on the margin of the SVM are called *support vectors*. These are usually comparatively few in number, and so are said to be *sparse*. And this is good, because it can be shown that the ultimate decision function for the SVM depends on *only* these, comparatively few, support vectors. It is equally important to keep in mind that these support vectors, those points serving to define the decision boundary, are not necessarily *typical* points: they may be far from the mean value of each of the two groups. On the other hand, sparsity can also be obtained using machines not belonging to the SVM family; see, for example, Biau (2010).

3.9 Neural networks

Neural networks (also called *artificial neural networks* or simply *neural nets*) define a huge class of nonlinear statistical models, yet the most basic components of this scheme are themselves linear models. This mixing of technologies leads to especially flexible and rich models. The essential idea is this: combine multiple, small models into a single large one, using links between the small models. The small models are often just linear regression models, and the links are formed in two stages. First, the output of the small model is transformed, using a so-called *transfer function*; such transfer functions can be quite complex themselves. Second, the output from the transformed small models is added together, in a weighted sum. Finally, this process can be repeated: multiple, new small models can be combined in multiple distinct weighted sums, where the entire collection of such intermediate sums is called a *hidden layer* in the network. In fact, a typical implementation of neural nets uses only one hidden layer.

Intricate model construction such as this is part of a larger mathematical approach to statistical learning called *generalized additive models*. It can be shown that such models, including neural nets, are extremely rich in the sense that they can approximate any dataset arbitrarily well, given enough hidden layers. Also, the transfer function in these schemes can be very simple or very complex; see DGL (chapter 30).

With the many weights and sequences of connected inputs and outputs in the several hidden layers, the model soon begins to look like a network of neurons and their synapses, hence its originating name. Whether or not a neuron model for statistical learning is valid, *because* it appears to mimic a biological process, is subject to debate: see our discussion in Section 2.9 on a possible taxonomy for learning machines. What is undeniable though is that such models, built of many tightly linked tiny pieces, are very flexible and capable of fitting any continuous outcome, given sufficient data and layers. Extreme model richness comes with the usual price: excellent fit for the given data and poor fit on new data. Otherwise expressed, neural nets historically were widely applied, until overfitting was identified as a routine problem. A more moderated appraisal is that properly applied, with sufficient validation, neural nets can be very accurate prediction schemes. As discussed in DGL (chapter 30), it is necessary to constrain the growth of the neurons (the nodes in each hidden layer) as the data is collected: the alternative will usually be a neural network that massively overfits the data.

3.10 Boosting

When looking for the structure in data one does not always have to construct the single, best possible description, or the single, best possible rule for predicting future outcomes. In many cases using a simple method, involving just one, or very few of the predictors can produce significantly more accurate results than complex models. One can then imagine constructing many such simple, easy-to-find rules and combining them to produce an accurate prediction rule. The boosting approach takes this one step further, by using a very simple base classifier repeatedly, each time on a different version of the data. It is this version-changing idea that is at the heart of the boosting scheme, now known to be among the best classifiers for many problems. The idea is simple: when a weighted sum of the simple rules misclassifies a data point, attach a higher weight to that point and apply the simple rule again. Repeatedly revising the weights on each data point, and changing the weights on each simple model, and finally summing over the simple rules leads the scheme to focus on the hardest-to-classify data points.

Recently it has been shown, on the other hand, that repeating the reweighting process indefinitely will often lead to overfitting in an interesting way: extreme iterations will lead to more or less *perfect* fitting of the given training data, and still provide good results on new data. Using VC dimension results (see Chapter 2), it is also known that boosting (with some help from so-called regularization) is an excellent performer; see Blanchard *et al.* (2003). This data reweighting scheme works with any simple rule, and boosting schemes can use truly very simple rules: for example, a tree having exactly one split, with two terminal nodes. The theory behind the boosting engine, however, does not itself require a simple base rule, and hence one can *boost* over big trees, linear models, logistic regression models, and more.

That is, one can take any base scheme and boost it, with the provable possibility that the result will be at least as good as the original, base classifier.

A recent, very thorough presentation of boosting, with discussion, begins here (Bartlett *et al.*, 2004) and continues with Koltchinskii and Yu (2004), Jiang (2004), Zhang (2004), Lugosi and Vayatis (2004). Mease *et al.* (2007, 2008) has a long and thoughtful discussion about the version of boosting called *logitboost*. Recall also the issues raised in Note 5 at the end of Chapter 2.

3.11 Evolutionary and genetic algorithms

Evolutionary algorithms, or *genetic algorithms*, are another family of biologically motivated methods, in this respect similar to neural networks (discussed above). Thus, each computational solution is viewed as a solution to a particular biological population problem, considered as a matter of "genetic fitness." They seek their inspiration from the way evolution "finds" the solutions and optimizes the performance of an individual or species: by means of replication (reproduction), slight random modifications (mutation), and the selection of the best-performing algorithms (survival of the fittest). In still other words, the scheme is "breeding" the best solutions and algorithms.

For all versions of these algorithms it is important to note that they are basically parametric equation-solving engines: they search a collection (possibly very large) of parameter values to find an optimal value. Hence they do not by themselves make predictions or classify, and are required to be linked to a particular prediction scheme. Equally important is that the problem must first be organized or *represented* as a parameter solution problem.

How this is done is a choice of the researcher, and the choice of the representation may significantly impact the resulting solution. More simply, a genetic algorithm can just as well use the apparent error of a model fit as a figure of merit; see, for example, Miller *et al.* (2003).

Yet, while it is not clear when a specific evolutionary fitness approach may be valid for making a prediction for a specific dataset, a mismatch between justification and successful classification need not be an obstacle in itself. Indeed, the evolutionary approach to parameter estimation, as a statistical problem, does not have some of the technical drawbacks of more familiar computational schemes. For much more on this topic, including an updated discussion of what might be called *computational evolution*; see Walker and Miller (2008), Banzhaf *et al.* (2006).

Notes

(1) A very comprehensive machine learning text is Hastie *et al.* (2009).

(2) Equations and complex mathematical devices are often critical for deep understanding of these prediction engines, as is gasoline in the engine of a car, yet in order to drive a car we don't need precise knowledge of the octane number or the problem of engine ignition timing.

(3) A recent study questions whether learning machines have led to *any* real progress over simple linear models: see Hand (2006) (with Comments and Rejoinder). It is difficult here to summarize the arguments, counter-arguments, and counter-counter-arguments presented there. In fact, we don't think this is a very interesting line of reasoning anyway. For one thing, the problem with benchmarking methods to find universal winners is provably mistaken: see Section 2.11. And more constructively, we take the position that relatively simple linear methods have a crucial role as interpretable reference models, applied *after* a much more complex learning machine has found (any) key predictive features in the data. Viewed in this light, linear models have a natural pairing with machine methods – each needs the other, each can inform the other in unexpected ways; see Section 5.11.

4

Three examples and several machines

A ship in harbor is safe – but that is not what ships are for.

John Shedd

4.1 Introduction

In this chapter we apply several learning machines to three datasets. These examples show some of the range, strengths, and pitfalls of the machines. The datasets include those connected to two published studies, concerning lupus and stroke; see König *et al.* (2007, 2008), Ward *et al.* (2006, 2009). We also study an artificially created file of cholesterol data. This data was generated using known cardiac health factors; see Note 1.

Regarding methods, we begin with two linear schemes, logistic regression and linear discriminant, and apply them to the cholesterol data. Then we apply four learning machine methods – k-nearest neighbor, boosting, Random Forests, and neural nets – with several variations, to all three datasets.

Our goal in this chapter is to see how these learning machines operate on real, or nearly real, data. We evaluate the machines using methods such as *out-of-bag resampling*, techniques which are described more fully later; see Chapter 10. Other methods also make brief appearances, simply as part of the standard learning machine toolkit.

It is not our intention to declare a single winner among these machine methods over all three datasets. Theory tells us that there is no hope of finding a single machine that is provably better than all others for all datasets: the "super-classifier" does not exist. It is also true that many methods are provably optimal, considered individually, when tuned properly and given sufficient data. Moreover, techniques called *ensemble methods* (see Chapter 12), which bring multiple, often very diverse, machines together into voting pools, can sharply improve prediction when compared with any of the individual machines in the pool. But this is also true: no amount of crafty tuning or sly voting transforms a single untuned machine, or collection of machines, from good into perfect for every dataset. Perfection can exist within certain families, but this ideal machine may be quite hard to locate in the family. For more details on this from theory, see Section 2.10.

Though real data is generally a better challenge to a given machine than artificial data, a simple artificial dataset allows us:

(1) to describe important statistical measures used for characterizing the performance of a particular learning machine when we are in complete charge of the mechanism generating the data;
(2) to use data that reveals important operating characteristics of learning machines, traits that are not so obvious from the equations and computer code driving them.

The two real-world examples, the lupus and stroke studies, are both oriented toward using learning machines for predicting patient outcomes within a large scale medical study. We start by describing the three datasets in more detail.

4.2 Simulated cholesterol data

Motivated by medical literature on the risk of developing coronary disease driven by high total cholesterol, we generated a simple dataset with only two variables, or features: the concentrations of low-density lipoprotein (LDL), and high-density lipoprotein (HDL); see Note 2. With just two features to work with we can display the results (predictions) of machines in a simple plot.

For the purposes of our simulated study, a person is *at risk* of developing coronary disease if any one of these conditions is true:

(1) total cholesterol (LDL+HDL) is greater than 240 mg/dL; *or*
(2) HDL is less than 35 mg/dL; *or*
(3) the ratio LDL/HDL is greater than 4.

Though they are motivated by medical research, these specific thresholds are chosen solely to allow for the illustration of learning machine concepts; see

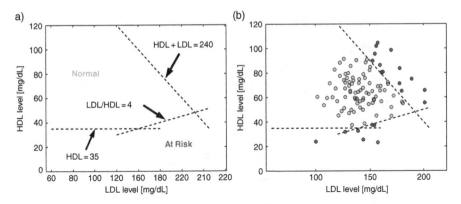

Figure 4.1   (a) The decision boundaries for the cholesterol data. (b) An instance of simulated data for the cholesterol problem. Light gray circles are not-at-risk subjects; dark gray circles are at-risk subjects.

Note 2. Each threshold defines a clear decision boundary between the healthy population (negatives) and those at risk (positives). In real-world medical diagnostic such sharp boundaries, jointly, would themselves function as the learning machine for making predictions.

Together the three conditions form an irregular decision boundary, plotted as a dotted line in Figure 4.1(a) and in all figures in this chapter. The dotted lines represent the hidden structure that learning machines are asked to find. Figure 4.1(b) shows a typical data sample.

Decision boundaries in real datasets are likely to be very complicated.

(1) The list of features can number in the thousands or millions, so the data often lives in some very high-dimensional space and the decision boundary cannot easily be visualized.
(2) The decision boundaries are usually not straight lines (or, in higher dimensions, even planes or "hyperplanes"). The boundaries between at risk and not at risk may be more complex than a single threshold, and more gradual rather than sharp.
(3) The regions defining risk are not necessarily connected; at-risk groups can be separated into many distinct regions, each with complex boundaries, with healthy subjects containing islands of at-risk subjects.
(4) Many biomedical decision functions and boundaries are often generated by combining scores from distinct medical tests, and our next two examples, stroke and lupus, illustrate this. The Barthel Index is such a

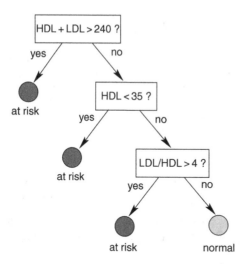

Figure 4.2   The decision tree corresponding to the decision boundaries for the cholesterol data.

summary score in the stroke dataset, as are the two comorbidity scores used in the lupus dataset.

(5) In this cholesterol data the three decision boundaries are binary (above/ below) and were specified by us. We can display this ideal decision tree from the three cut-points; see Figure 4.2. Cut-points in real-world decision trees are estimated from the data; see Chapter 6.

(6) In an effort to bring the cholesterol data back to a more realistic setting we have, in addition to the simple, sharp boundary dataset, simulated *fuzzy* cholesterol data for which the decision boundaries are not sharp. This fuzziness is introduced using a probability algorithm; see Note 3. The fuzzy boundaries are displayed in Figure 4.3(a) and sample data from this fuzzy scheme is displayed in Figure 4.3(b).

We generate two cholesterol datasets as follows. Dataset 1 will be used to *train* various learning machines, meaning we will use that file to develop and construct models. Dataset 2 will be used to *test* the models constructed using dataset 1. Dataset 2 is statistically independent of dataset 1, but was drawn from the same larger population as dataset 1 (by being simulated and using the same mechanism, in this case). Similarly, dataset 3 generated using the fuzzy mechanism is used to develop models for that data, while dataset 4 will be used to test them.

The concepts of *training* and *testing* will be used throughout the text.

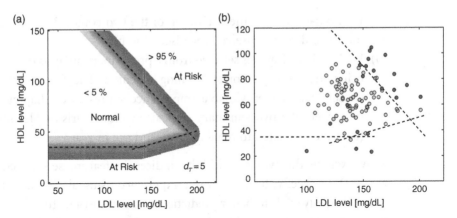

Figure 4.3   (a) The boundary for the fuzzy cholesterol data. A probabilistic algorithm was used to soften the decision boundary; see Note 1 for details. (b) An instance of simulated data using the probabilistic fuzzy boundary algorithm.

4.3 Lupus data

The source database for our lupus analyses includes all patients diagnosed with systemic lupus erythematosus (SLE) and hospitalized in California from 1996 to 2000; see Ward *et al.* (2006). During this period all acute-care, non-federal hospitals in California provided anonymized patient data, including age, gender, race, principal diagnosis, discharge diagnosis, and insurance type.

Of the more than 20,000 patients with SLE who were hospitalized during these years, 3839 patients had at least one unscheduled hospitalization for which the principal diagnosis was SLE. Of these 3839, 109 died during the first such hospitalization. Our first analysis, Lupus A, uses death during the first hospitalization as the outcome (dependent) variable, for the $N = 3839$ patients.

The principal diagnosis for each subject was SLE, and candidates for predictor variables were age, sex, race, insurance type, a series of yes/no flags indicating the presence of 41 conditions upon discharge, and two summary measures derived from the diagnosis flags, the Charlson Index and the SLE Comorbidity Index. From these features, we selected three subgroups for analysis.

(1) BIGSET: All 34 features identified as *possibly* relevant by the clinicians, except the two comorbidity indices, Charlson and SLE comorbidity.
(2) MOSTIMP: Twelve features identified by clinicians as *probably* most important, including age, the yes/no flag for respiratory failure, and all

yes/no flags used in the derivation of the two comorbidity indices (but not the indices themselves; see discussion below).

(3) RFIMP: Four features selected from a preliminary analysis of all features using the Random Forest learning machine. The features that were chosen had higher variable importance scores (see Chapter 7) and these were the two summary clinical indicies Charlson, Slecomb, rfail (a predictor related to renal failure), and age in years.

Why exclude the two comorbidity indices in feature sets BIGSET and MOSTIMP? Briefly, because in our experience using all available features at least initially leads to better predictions. Sometimes a feature can increase the computational demand in a learning machine analysis, leading to lengthy run times: pulling out noisy and less informative features beforehand can be less expensive in the long run. Also, features in a very complete list can compete directly with or mask the most useful features. The two comorbidity indices are linear functions of the original yes/no flags. It is possible that *locally* an index is a better predictor than other combinations of features or simple functions of the data, for example, for younger female patients. However, using a set of separate features, each of which in itself may be a less effective predictor, can lead to better overall prediction, better than using a derived feature alone or in combination with its components.

4.4 Stroke data

The third dataset is from a prospective study of survival and recovery following a stroke, for 1754 patients from 23 neurology departments in Germany in 1998 and 1999; see König *et al.* (2007, 2008). As described there, the Barthel Index (BI) was used to classify recovery for patients surviving to 100 days (with a window of 90–150 days) as complete or incomplete. The BI ranges from 0 to 100 with higher scores indicating better functional independence; for background see Mahoney and Barthel (1965).

To develop prognostic models for survival and functional recovery, patients were assigned to one of three categories:

(1) alive with complete functional recovery (BI of 95 or higher);
(2) alive with incomplete functional recovery (BI less than 95);
(3) not alive (BI assigned value of −10).

The stroke data was systematically analyzed in König *et al.* (2007, 2008). Here we conduct a reanalysis and study the two datasets in the original analysis. The first, which we label Stroke A, includes the patients who were alive at the endpoint (categories 1 and 2), and uses the BI functional recovery score as the outcome variable: a total of 1754 patients, with 1156 having complete recovery, and 598 incomplete recovery (or death).

The second dataset, labeled Stroke B, includes a separately collected group of patients, and also uses BI as the outcome score to be predicted. The complex, careful strategy behind this data collection is detailed in König *et al.* (2007). In particular, the Stroke-B patients came from clinics and cardiac centers not involved in the Stroke-A data collection, so these patients are expected to be a more stringent, realistic test of the machines generated using Stroke A.

As with the lupus dataset there were many potential predictors in the two stroke datasets. The study authors (König *et al.*, 2007, 2008) used a preliminary Random Forest analysis, expert medical opinion, and other more classical statistical techniques to select 11 features for in-depth analysis. For more of the medical background see Bonita and Beaglehole (1988). They selected several yes/no variables (neurological complications, fever > 38°C, localization to the anterior cerebral artery, localization to the lenticulostriate arteries, prior stroke, and gender); continuous or near-continuous variables (age and NIH Stroke Scale score at admission); and two categorical components of the NIH Stroke Scale (motor left arm and motor right arm, each coded 0 = no drift, to 4 = no movement). Below we reanalyze this data using these two sets of predictors: that selected by König *et al.* using a variety of advanced classical methods, = REDUCED, and the full list of predictors with no preselection, = FULL.

4.5 Biomedical *means* unbalanced

It is important to observe that, in each of the three datasets we look at here, the number of subjects in the two outcome groups is not the same. Statisticians will say these three datasets are *unbalanced*, while the machine learning community uses the term *imbalanced*.

It is very common in biomedical studies that there are fewer patients in the at-risk group than are normals. Such data is often less of a problem for computer-science-driven analysis of learning machine performance. However, severely unbalanced data also occurs in many non-medical contexts: the evaluation of credit-worthiness is of this type, as there are many more truly credit-worthy individuals than there are not so worthy.

Such data can undermine the construction of a machine, as well as subvert any estimates for the error rate of a machine. Briefly, the problem is that a very large group of survivors and a tiny group of nonsurvivors can suggest to any machine that the best bet is on *survive*. And if only two out of 100 patients do not survive then we seemingly make only a 2% error by declaring all cases to be *survive*. But this ignores the distinction between the two outcomes, and the costs of making a wrong decision. How to deal with this problem of unbalanced data is discussed in more detail in Chapter 11.

An important warning: We recommend using some balancing plan *always* except when the groups are close in size. These plans are usually easy to implement, and there is no good reason for not doing so; see Chapter 11.

A quick, if indirect, way to check for machine performance in the presence of unbalanced data is to evaluate the sensitivity and specificity of the method, and for this see Section 4.6.

4.6 Measures of machine performance

Before presenting the results of learning machines on these datasets we must first describe methods for characterizing the performance of these machines. Full details on error rates and error estimation are given in Chapter 11.

Basic statistical measures of performance of any learning machine (or any diagnostic or statistical decision-making) are *sensitivity*, *specificity*, and the *overall error rate* and *precision*.

Sensitivity measures the fraction of truly at-risk subjects correctly identified among the group identified as "positives" by the learning machine. It tells us how well the machine finds the at-risk subjects.

Specificity measures the fraction of healthy people correctly identified among the group identified as "negatives" by the machine. It tells us how specific we are when we declare someone not at risk. Specificity helps guard against declaring someone at risk who really isn't at risk.

These two measures, sensitivity and specificity, are coupled in the following sense: we could identify every truly at risk subject by declaring *all* subjects to be at risk, but then we would also be incorrectly naming many healthy subjects as at risk. Similarly, if we identify no subjects as at risk then we never make the mistake of misclassifying a healthy subject, but then we're never catching *any* at-risk subject. Either approach is extreme and costly.

Both these measures are important to report, but we also need a global measure of the performance of a machine. For this, we use the *overall error*, the fraction of incorrect classifications among all subjects, in either direction. The overall error is the number of at-risk subjects declared by the machine to be healthy, plus the number of healthy subjects declared to be at risk, divided by the total sample. The overall error rate gives us an estimate of the probability of making an error on new data.

As discussed in Chapter 10, there are statistical problems engendered in calculating the performance of a machine on just the dataset on which it was constructed (trained), and then using that as an estimate of its presumed performance on new data. However, there is now a large library of good methods available for avoiding some of these statistical problems.

One of these methods is the out-of-bag sampling method, *OOB*. Briefly, it operates this way. Select from the given dataset a fraction of all the data. This can be a selection that uses replacement, where each subject and associated predictors are returned to the dataset after each draw. This is a *bootstrap resampling method*. It is also possible to use sampling that does not use replacement, in which case a random fraction, say 75%, of the subjects are selected.

In either case, the sampled data is used to train the machine (generate a model) and the data *not* selected in the random sample is used to test the machine.

We apply the OOB method to the lupus and stroke data: this is a good default method for real data. For real-world data a sensible plan for getting good error estimates is therefore:

(1) draw a random sample from the data, using replacement, or a simple fraction of the data;
(2) train a machine on the sampled data;
(3) test the machine on the data not drawn (the OOB sample);
(4) repeat steps (1), (2), and (3) many times (say, 1000);
(5) taking the average of sensitivity, specificity, and overall error from (1), (2), and (3) gives the OOB estimate of each error value;

(6) finally, the machine that is generated using all the data is the reported one, and the OOB errors are its measures of performance.

As the cholesterol data is itself simulated, we can apply the OOB method and also create (simulate) new examples of the data. This allows us the rare luxury of seeing how well the real-world applicable OOB method does, at least on this data. We pursue this in Chapter 10.

4.7 Linear analysis of cholesterol data

We start with the linear discriminant analysis and logistic regression methods that are very commonly used in biological studies. In both methods the decision boundary is linear, a single line or plane, which is specified mathematically as a weighted combination of the individual features (independent variables).

As discussed in Chapter 5, logistic regression also generates an estimate of the probability that a subject belongs to one group or another. For now, let's note that estimating this probability of group membership is very definitely not the same as classifying a subject into one group or another.

The dashed lines are the actual decision boundaries as in Figure 4.4(a) and (b). We've used shading to describe the fuzzy boundary in Figure 4.5(a) and (b).

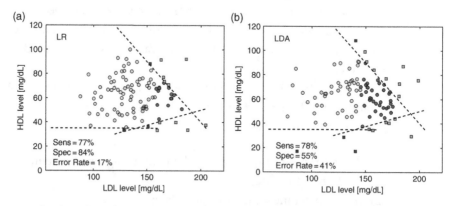

Figure 4.4   Application of two linear methods to the cholesterol data: (a) logistic regression; (b) linear discriminant. Light gray boxes are at-risk patients correctly classified as at risk; dark gray boxes are at-risk patients misclassified as not at risk; light gray circles are not-at-risk patients correctly classified as not at risk; dark gray circles are not-at-risk patients misclassified as at risk.

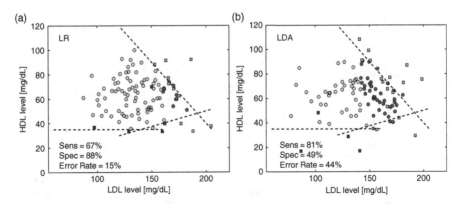

Figure 4.5   Application of two linear methods to the cholesterol data with the fuzzy (soft) boundary: (a) logistic regression; (b) linear discriminant. Key as in Figure 4.4

The figures show that the real decision boundary for the cholesterol data requires *three* straight lines to delineate at-risk subjects from healthy subjects. Therefore we would not expect linear discriminant or logistic regression to perform well since both are purely linear methods, that is, linear in the original measurements.

In these figures, the light gray circles and dark gray squares represent correctly identified healthy and at-risk subjects. The light gray squares are false positives (healthy subjects identified by the machine as at risk), and the dark gray circles are false negatives (at-risk subjects declared by the machine to be healthy); together they are the errors, or misclassifications. The abundance of light gray squares and dark gray circles reflects the weak decision power of these two linear methods for the cholesterol data. The values of overall error, sensitivity, and specificity are given in all figures (Figure 4.4(a) and (b), Figure 4.5(a) and (b)).

4.8 Nonlinear analysis of cholesterol data

Given the not very inspiring results above, we see that more flexible, alternative methods should be tried on the cholesterol data. One generally excellent method is a *decision tree* (see Chapter 6). Briefly, a decision tree repeatedly divides up (partitions) the data and defines a new decision boundary for each partition. Each decision boundary may be simple or complex. The tree method "sees" the data only very locally; it does not presume that the true decision boundary for the dataset is a *single* straight line or plane, or any curved surface for that matter.

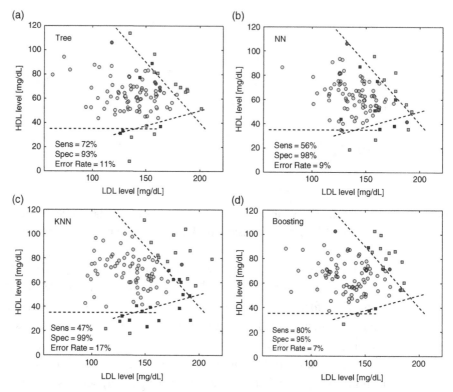

Figure 4.6   Application of four other learning machines to the cholesterol data: (a) a single decision tree; (b) a neural network with 20 hidden nodes in one layer; (c) k-nearest neighbors with $k = 5$; (d) boosting on stumps (two-node decision trees at each iteration) with 500 iterations. Key as in Figure 4.4.

DGL (chapter 20) presents a full range of alternatives for how a dataset might be carved up in a decision tree approach.

In Figure 4.6 we display the performances of a single tree approach and three other learning machines:

(a) a single, possibly very large, decision tree;
(b) a single-layer neural network with 20 hidden units;
(c) a k-nearest-neighbor scheme with the number of neighbors $k = 5$;
(d) a boosting scheme using two-node trees (so-called stumps) as base classifiers and run with 500 iterations.

All of these methods have lower *overall* error than the linear methods we just studied, but the inequality between sensitivity and specificity in each highlights the problem of unbalanced data; see Section 4.5. But how, in biomedical terms, is each machine making its decisions, and what can the machines tell us about the disease process? And how can we "tune" or improve the action of any of these machines?

For example, a support vector machine can use a variety of different so-called *kernels*, among which are linear, polynomial, and so-called radial basis functions kernels. To use a kernel, we may need to select machine parameters and assign values to some of them. Parameter selection and assignment is often not a matter of finding slightly better decision rules, and in these cases we are not fine-tuning a model, we are making or breaking it. Figure 4.7 shows three different instances of a support vector machine (SVM) producing rather similar results, but these were obtained only after labor-intensive optimization; see Note 4.

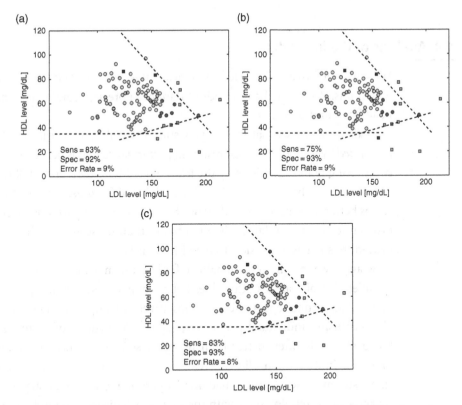

Figure 4.7   Application of three versions of a support vector machine using (a) linear kernel, (b) cubic kernel, and (c) radial basis functions kernel.

There is, therefore, a problem with pursuing a path of extensive tuning and parameter selection: given a wide library of possible variants for a type of machine, it can be hard to verify that the variant ultimately selected does truly improve on all the other variants. Selecting wisely from within a class of machines, for example, selecting a single SVM with a particular type of kernel, is an ongoing area of research in the machine learning community; see DGL (chapter 18). As with more familiar statistical techniques, it is usually true that the more data we have, the easier it is to know that we have used the optimal learning machine. But note that finding excellent families of learning machines is a well-studied problem and has many fine solutions. Finding an excellent machine within a given family is usually the truly hard problem.

Let's move on to the authentic, real-world examples.

4.9 Analysis of the lupus data

We next study two real-world biomedical datasets, lupus and stroke, starting with lupus. We apply the methods of Random Forests, neural nets, k-nearest neighbors, and boosting.

In Figure 4.8 we see that applying boosting, to a collection of features, RFIMP, *preselected* by Random Forests, results in performance that is between the other two starting points, that is using the feature sets MOSTIMP and BIGSET.

Note especially that starting with the full list of features, given in BIGSET, seems better in terms of overall error, than using either shorter list. Using the original features in a dataset is often better than preselection when using a procedure such as a decision tree or Random Forest.

So again we see this general pattern for learning machines. Starting from a complete list of features often does better than starting from a preselected, filtered list. And to repeat, there is a closely related, important idea that is less obvious: using individual predictors, separately, instead of forming combined scores, is often better than using those scores. There is certainly a practical, indeed often clinical, reason for preferring a more convenient, single summary score, but a machine – operating as a pure binary decision-maker – can often do better with the raw data. This issue is studied in more detail in the context of single decision trees; see Chapter 6.

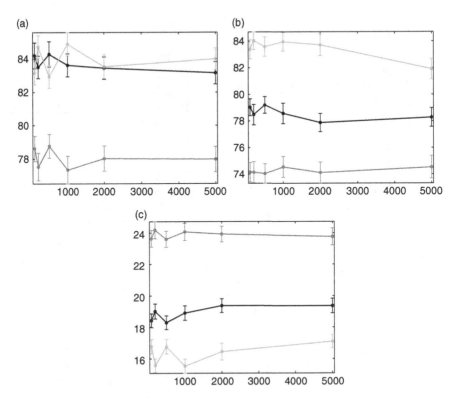

Figure 4.8   Random Forests applied to the lupus data. Performance is measured in terms of (a) sensitivity, (b) specificity, and (c) overall error. Three different sets of features were sent to the program: BIGSET = dark gray line, RFIMP = black line, MOSTIMP = light gray line; see text for descriptions of these feature sets. The x-axis gives the number of trees grown in each forest, and the error bars are one standard deviation across 100 OOB runs.

In Figure 4.9 neural networks were applied with varying numbers of hidden nodes, we again see that the full list BIGSET seems to do better than the preselected lists, RFIMP and MOSTIMP.

Observe that the performance of the neural nets *on average* seems similar to that of Random Forests. Theory on neural nets reports that with enough nodes and hidden layers data having *any* distribution can be well modeled. However, note the very large error bars for this method. At every selection of number of nodes, the OOB results are extremely variable. Finally, theory explains that good modeling does not require

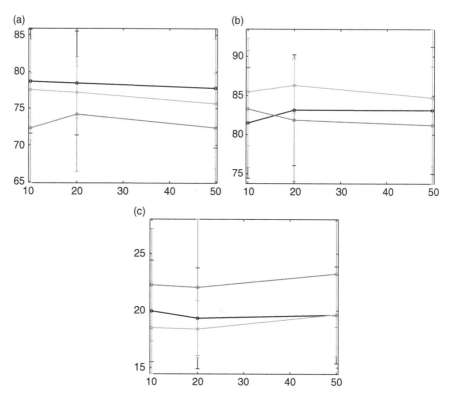

Figure 4.9   Neural networks applied to the lupus data. Performance is measured in terms of
(a) sensitivity, (b) specificity, and (c) overall error. As in Figure 4.8, three different
sets of features were sent to the program: BIGSET = dark gray line , RFIMP = black
line, MOSTIMP = light gray line; see text for descriptions of these feature sets. The
x-axis records the number of nodes in the single hidden layer, and the error bars are
one standard deviation across 100 OOB runs.

arbitrarily large neural networks in terms of layers: at most two hidden
layers are required for good modeling; see DGL (chapter 30). It is possible,
as well, that more layers might stabilize the performance of the neural
networks, but this is a subject for further research.

In Figure 4.10 the performance of the k-nearest neighbors seems highly
dependent on k, the number of neighbors in the analysis, and the error bars
seem large, compared to Random Forests, but not large compared to neural
networks. Using the classification method with fewer neighbors seems to
work better for this data.

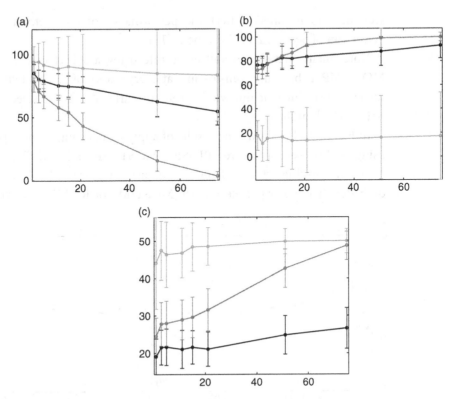

Figure 4.10   *k*-Nearest neighbors applied to the lupus data. Performance is measured in terms of (a) sensitivity, (b) specificity, and (c) overall error. As in Figure 4.8, three different sets of features were sent to the program: BIGSET = dark gray line, RFIMP = black line, MOSTIMP = light gray line; see text for descriptions of these feature sets. The *x*-axis records the number, *k*, of neighbors used in each run, and the error bars are one standard deviation across 100 OOB runs.

One problem with large *k*, compared to the size of the data, is that in classifying each new data point, the machine is asked to report back about its local neighborhood, but if *local* becomes too large then it stops being local. Using an average over a very large subset of the data (using *k* large) is a scheme that puts each new data point in one group or the other based on basically just the group sizes, and the sensitivity rates, in particular, drop steadily as *k* increases.

Recall our often-stated mantra: *Information is local.* The phenomenon operating here is also confirmed by theory: selection of *k* needs to grow as the size of the data, but not too fast. Letting *k* grow while fixing the sample size is seen here to negatively affect the performance of the method. See the discussion of Section 2.11, Comment (12).

Note finally that the overall error rate using a subset of the features, MOSTIMP, is basically coin-tossing, at every choice of k. This tells us that not every learning machine would prefer to start with a list preselected using only clinical intuition.

In Figure 4.11 is shown the results of applying boosting to the lupus data using all three sets of features, BIGSET, MOSTIMP, and RFIMP.

For this machine starting from the full list of features, BIGSET, seems to do better than either preselected list, MOSTIMP or RFIMP. The error bars

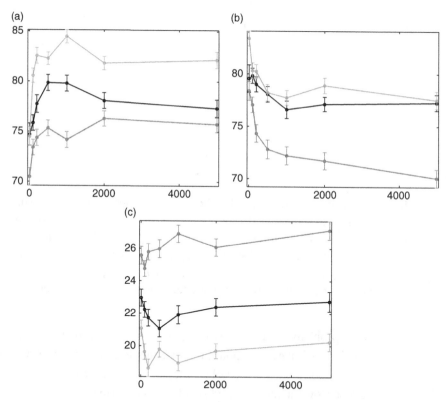

Figure 4.11   Boosting applied to the lupus data. Performance is measured in terms of (a) sensitivity, (b) specificity, and (c) overall error. As in Figure 4.8, three different sets of features were sent to the program: BIGSET = dark gray line, RFIMP = black line, MOSTIMP = light gray line; see text for descriptions of these feature sets. The x-axis records the number of iterations (the number of boosting steps), and the error bars are one standard deviation across 100 OOB runs.

are respectable and the method is relatively stable across the number of boosting iterations.

4.10 Analysis of the stroke data

Moving on to the Stroke-A data, we can inspect Figures 4.12, 4.13, 4.14, and 4.15.

As shown in Figure 4.12, Random Forests was given two different starter lists of features: REDUCE, which was derived using a variety of statistical methods to preselect the features, as described in König *et al.* (2007, 2008),

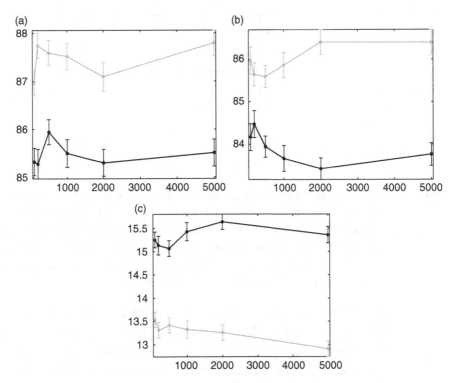

Figure 4.12 Random Forests applied to the Stroke-A data. Performance is measured in terms of (a) sensitivity, (b) specificity, and (c) overall error. Two sets of predictors were used: the dark gray line is the performance for Random Forests applied to FULL, using the complete list of predictors for the stroke data; the black line is the performance for Random Forests applied to REDUCE, a smaller feature list derived using a variety of methods as discussed in König *et al.* (2007, 2008). The *x*-axis records the number of trees grown, and the error bars are one standard deviation across 100 OBB runs.

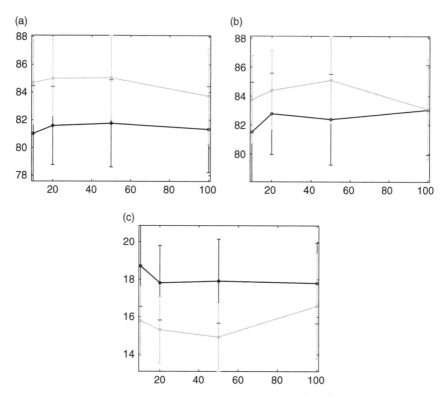

Figure 4.13   Neural networks applied to the Stroke-A data. Performance is measured in terms of (a) sensitivity, (b) specificity, and (c) overall error. As in Figure 4.12, the dark gray line is the performance of the method as applied to FULL, the complete feature list, and the black line is the performance of the method as applied to REDUCE, a preselected smaller feature list. The x-axis records the number of hidden nodes, and the error bars are one standard deviation across 100 OOB runs.

and FULL, which was the original and complete list of features for this data. The improvement resulting from starting with the full list is dramatic, and the error rate here is smaller than that reported in the König papers.

Neural networks applied to the Stroke-A data are given in Figure 4.13. Despite the low averaged error rate, the extremely wide error bars, at every choice of number of nodes, make any practical interpretation or use of this method problematic.

As shown in Figure 4.14, the method of k-nearest neighbors appears to do rather well when using only a handful of neighbors, and $k = 1$ seems to do quite well in fact, when the errors are averaged over 100 OOB runs. As with

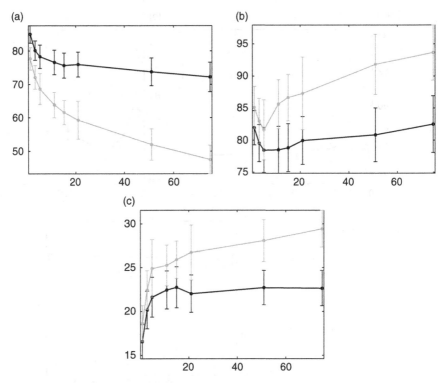

Figure 4.14   *k*-Nearest neighbors applied to the Stroke-A data. Performance is measured in terms of (a) sensitivity, (b) specificity, and (c) overall error. As in Figure 4.12, the dark gray line is the performance of the method as applied to FULL, the complete feature list, and the black line is the performance of the method as applied to REDUCE, a preselected smaller feature list. The *x*-axis records *k*, the number of nearest neighbors used, and the error bars are one standard deviation across 100 OOB runs.

neural networks, the error bars are a problem, especially at the higher number of neighbors.

Boosting analysis, as shown in Figure 4.15, uses the program BoosTexter; see Appendix A1 for details.

Next, the results of the four machines, Random Forests, boosting, neural nets, and *k*-nearest neighbors, as applied to Stroke B, are shown in Figures 4.16, 4.17, 4.18, and 4.19. The output from these methods on Stroke B runs closely parallel to those we've seen for Stroke-A data.

Not explored here is the interesting possibility that training any machine on Stroke-A data and then testing it on Stroke-B data may, or

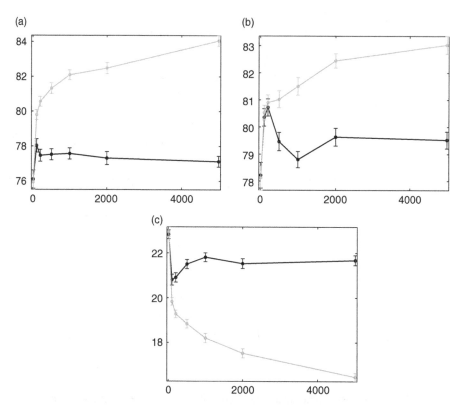

Figure 4.15 Boosting applied to the Stroke-A data. Performance is measured in terms of (a) sensitivity, (b) specificity, and (c) overall error. As in Figure 4.12, the dark gray line is the performance of the method as applied to FULL, the complete feature list, and the black line is the performance of the method as applied to REDUCE, a preselected smaller feature list. The x-axis records k, the number of boosting iterations used, and the error bars are one standard deviation across 100 OOB runs.

may not, return the same error rates, and the reverse is possible. The two datasets, as discussed in König *et al.* (2007, 2008), are similar but collected at different places and separate times. Indeed, a central reason for collecting the two stroke datasets was to examine the prognostic differences in differently collected data. Moreover, *if* the error rates, and stability across user-parameter settings, error bars, etc., were determined to be basically equivalent then we should consider pooling the data in a Stroke-A+B dataset and training the better-performing machine on that data.

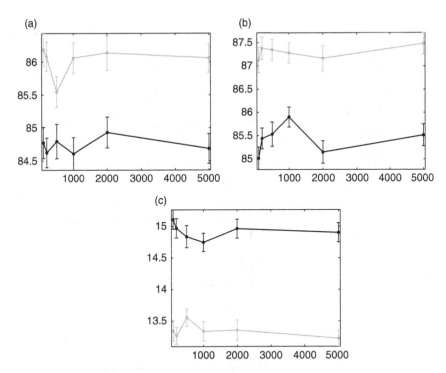

Figure 4.16   Random Forests applied to Stroke-B data. Performance is measured in terms of (a) sensitivity, (b) specificity, and (c) overall error. As in Figure 4.12, the dark gray line is the performance of the method as applied to FULL, the complete feature list, and the black line is the performance of the method as applied to REDUCE, a preselected smaller feature list. The x-axis records k, the number of trees grown, and the error bars are one standard deviation across 100 OOB runs.

4.11 Further analysis of the lupus and stroke data

Let's pursue the analysis of our three datasets in more detail. Here we present results from intensive optimization of each of the machines. This will give us some sense of the lower limits for the error rates for each machine. In no case do we find error rates that are especially close to zero: there is no super-classifier in this lot.

The possibility of using two different methods for calculating errors is studied in Table 4.1.

The methods are OOB, where a sample is drawn from the data, a machine generated on the sample, and then tested on the data not sampled, and

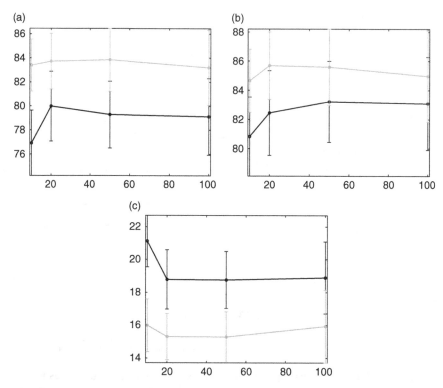

Figure 4.17   Neural networks applied to the Stroke-B data. Performance is measured in terms of (a) sensitivity, (b) specificity, and (c) overall error. As in Figure 4.12, the dark gray line is the performance of the method as applied to FULL, the complete feature list, and the black line is the performance of the method as applied to REDUCE, a preselected smaller feature list. The x-axis records the number of hidden nodes, and the error bars are one standard deviation across 100 OOB runs.

simulated, that is, replicated data. We normally don't have additional data just for testing, but for the cholesterol data we do. In this analysis a series of computer runs was done to attempt to optimize the performance of each machine, before the testing phase began using 100 OOB runs or 100 replications. Also, the OOB method was applied to balanced data, since the original code generating the data usually had many more normal subjects than at-risk subjects. But there was no balancing when the replicate method was used. There is evidently not much difference in using balanced, or not balanced, data on the results for sensitivity and specificity. Note that the linear discriminant method does not do very well: by construction, the data

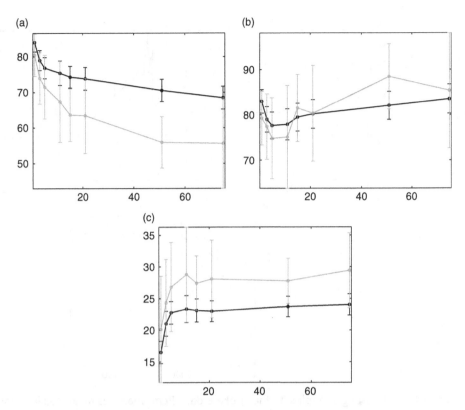

Figure 4.18   *k*-Nearest neighbors applied to the Stroke-B data. Performance is measured in terms of (a) sensitivity, (b) specificity, and (c) overall error. As in Figure 4.12, the dark gray line is the performance of the method as applied to FULL, the complete feature list, and the black line is the performance of the method as applied to REDUCE, a preselected smaller feature list. The *x*-axis records *k*, the number of nearest neighbors, and the error bars are one standard deviation across 100 OOB runs.

was not linear. On the other hand, the other methods are essentially the same in terms of error rates: nonlinearity doesn't seem to bother them greatly.

In Table 4.2 we study the consequences of using optimized methods, but as applied to the unbalanced lupus data.

As described earlier there are three different sets of features we could start with: BIGSET, with 34 features; MOSTIMP, a selection of 12 features thought most important by clinicians; and RFIMP, a selection of just four features, using a preliminary Random Forests run. The estimated error rates are essentially the same for all methods, but the

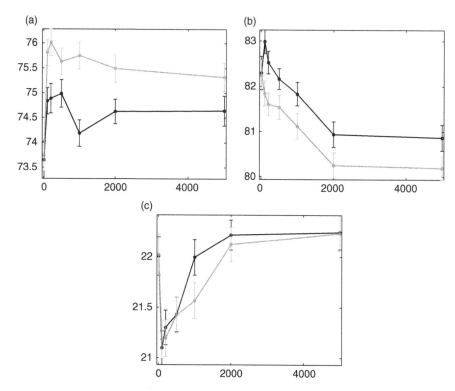

Figure 4.19   Boosting as applied to the Stroke-B data. Performance is measured in terms of
(a) sensitivity, (b) specificity, and (c) overall error. As in Figure 4.12, the dark gray
line is the performance of the method as applied to FULL, the complete feature list,
and the black line is the performance of the method as applied to REDUCE, a
preselected smaller feature list. The x-axis records the number of iterations used,
and the error bars are one standard deviation across 100 OOB runs.

sensitivity and specificity numbers point to the horrors of using very
unbalanced data for optimization and error estimation. Basically all the
machines work by declaring everyone healthy, that is, as having survived
the initial 72-hour stay in hospital. Intensive optimization does not necessarily overcome lack of balance.

Table 4.3 shows the more salutary effects of balancing the lupus data
before the optimization begins.

The effect of using a preselected group of features is also worthy of
note, and is mostly clearly seen by comparing the results of the
MOSTIMP and BIGSET feature list with those of the smallest, most

Table 4.1 Further analysis of the cholesterol data. The several methods were each optimized by intensive user-parameter tuning. For NN, 50 hidden nodes were used; for k-NN, k was chosen to be 5; for boosting, 100 iterations were done; for SVM, a radial basis function for the kernel was applied. The single decision tree had no adjustable parameters, and LDA used an unstructured covariance matrix. The error rates are essentially the same apart from the LDA method. Two methods for calculating the error rates were used; see Section 4.10

Machine	Error rate	Sensitivity	Specificity
	Monte Carlo		
NN	0.81 ± 0.42	96 ± 2	100
k-NN	1.6 ± 0.58	93 ± 3.2	100
Boosting	2.5 ± 0.59	89 ± 3.1	99 ± 0.4
SVM (RBF)	2.1 ± 0.65	89 ± 3.7	100
Single tree	3.4 ± 0.84	86 ± 3.7	99 ± 0.54
LDA	34 ± 2.2	82 ± 4.2	63 ± 2.4
	OOB (with balancing)		
NN	0.95 ± 2.2	97 ± 2.7	99 ± 3.5
k-NN	2.7 ± 1.2	92 ± 6.2	99 ± 0.9
Boosting	3.5 ± 1.5	89 ± 7.7	98 ± 1.5
SVM (RBF)	3.7 ± 1.5	82 ± 8.2	99 ± 1.1
Single tree	4.7 ± 1.8	85 ± 9.1	97 ± 1.4
LDA	34 ± 3.7	75 ± 7.2	64 ± 4.7

highly selected set, RFIMP. We see that as more features are added, the methods k-nearest neighbor (k-NN), support vector machine (SVM), and linear discriminant (LDA), all appear to suffer. On BIGSET, all three of these machines are essentially random coin-tossing, with error rates close to 50%.

Tables 4.4 and 4.5 show the results of optimizing the machines on the Stroke-A and Stroke-B datasets.

Recall that both of these are nearly balanced to start with. For neural networks (NN), 50 hidden nodes were chosen for best performance; for k-nearest neighbor (k-NN) $k = 1$, and for boosting 100 iterations were generated for each run. The results show that under this optimization Random Forests seems to do best, but it is competitive with k-NN. The

Table 4.2 Six machines applied to the unbalanced lupus dataset, using three different feature sets; see Section 4.3 for details. RFIMP has four features, MOSTIMP has 12 features, BIGSET has 26 features. All methods do quite well in terms of overall error rate, but note that sensitivity and specificity are very different, except for the linear discriminant method. Basically the machines are declaring most or all subjects as having survived the first 72-hour hospital stay: this group is much larger than the group that did not survive. The analysis calls out for balancing, for which see Table 4.3

Predictor set	Machine	Error rate	Sensitivity	Specificity
RFIMP	SVM	2.84 ± 0.38	0	100
	Boosting	2.9 ± 0.4	22 ± 6.4	99 ± 0.27
	k-NN	2.91 ± 0.35	6.1 ± 9.9	100
	NN	3.05 ± 0.38	14 ± 6.4	99 ± 0.33
	Single tree	3.72 ± 0.44	21 ± 6.4	98 ± 0.42
	LDA	23.53 ± 2.8	82 ± 5.7	76 ± 2.9
MOSTIMP	k-NN	2.82 ± 0.33	0.022 ± 0.22	100
	SVM	2.83 ± 0.34	0	100
	NN	3.01 ± 0.36	$0\,9.9 \pm 4.9$	99 ± 0.25
	Boosting	3.04 ± 0.37	14 ± 5.8	99 ± 0.3
	Single tree	3.87 ± 0.5	16 ± 6.4	98 ± 0.44
	LDA	38.11 ± 4.6	83 ± 9.9	61 ± 5
BIGSET	k-NN	2.79 ± 0.32	0	100
	SVM	2.81 ± 0.35	0	100
	LDA	2.84 ± 0.35	0	100
	Boosting	2.96 ± 0.33	21 ± 5.9	99 ± 0.29
	NN	3.04 ± 0.37	17 ± 6.4	99 ± 0.29
	Single tree	3.91 ± 0.49	22 ± 6.6	98 ± 0.51

single decision tree, boosting, and the SVM are comparable to each other and weaker performers than the others. LDA simply does not handle this data very well, and is virtually doing random coin-tossing, for both Stroke A and Stroke B. For all these machines the specificity and sensitivity for each are quite close, suggesting that any lack of balance in the data is not causing a problem in the later analysis.

Table 4.3 Seven machines, with same feature sets as in Table 4.2, but now the data has been balanced before being sent to the machines. Sensitivity and specificity are now more aligned. See Section 4.10 for more discussion of these results

Predictor set	Machine	Error rate	Sensitivity	Specificity
RFIMP	RF	18.3 ± 4.4	84 ± 7.6	79 ± 6.3
	k-NN	19.1 ± 4.8	85 ± 7.1	77 ± 7.2
	NN	19.3 ± 4.4	78 ± 7.1	83 ± 6.7
	Single tree	21.0 ± 5.1	81 ± 8.2	77 ± 8.3
	Boosting	21.1 ± 5.1	80 ± 8	78 ± 7.4
	SVM	28.1 ± 5.4	70 ± 10	74 ± 11
	LDA	29.7 ± 11	70 ± 12	70 ± 17
MOSTIMP	NN	22.0 ± 6	74 ± 7.8	82 ± 7.8
	RF	23.6 ± 4.6	79 ± 7.7	74 ± 7.4
	k-NN	24.5 ± 5	79 ± 8	72 ± 7.1
	Boosting	24.8 ± 4.8	73 ± 7.8	77 ± 7.4
	Single tree	26.7 ± 5.8	75 ± 9.4	72 ± 9.4
	SVM	45.6 ± 5.8	45 ± 17	63 ± 17
	LDA	48.8 ± 9.9	50 ± 15	52 ± 28
BIGSET	RF	15.5 ± 4.5	85 ± 7	84 ± 7
	NN	18.4 ± 2.5	77 ± 3.5	86 ± 6.5
	Boosting	18.6 ± 5.3	83 ± 7.9	80 ± 6.6
	Single tree	21.3 ± 4.8	81 ± 7.7	77 ± 8.4
	k-NN	44.1 ± 12	94 ± 12	18 ± 35
	SVM	45.6 ± 5.5	44 ± 14	65 ± 14
	LDA	50.8 ± 3.1	3 ± 12	97 ± 13

Table 4.4 Seven machines analyzing the Stroke-A data, with original data (top), and pre-balanced data (bottom). The machines are comparable in terms of their conclusions except for LDA, which is making only random coin tosses in its decision-making

Machine	Error rate	Sensitivity	Specificity
RF	15.1 ± 1.7	86 ± 2.6	84 ± 2.5
k-NN	16.6 ± 1.9	85 ± 2.6	82 ± 3.1
NN	17.8 ± 2.2	81 ± 3.1	83 ± 3
Single tree	20.5 ± 2.1	80 ± 3.2	79 ± 3.7

Table 4.4 (cont.)

Machine	Error rate	Sensitivity	Specificity
Boosting	20.8 ± 2.4	78 ± 3.8	80 ± 3.2
SVM	21.0 ± 1.9	76 ± 3.4	82 ± 3.3
LDA	51.8 ± 11	53 ± 22	44 ± 44
RF	12.9 ± 1.7	88 ± 2.7	86 ± 3
NN	14.9 ± 1.8	85 ± 3.1	85 ± 2.3
Boosting	16.5 ± 1.8	84 ± 3.1	83 ± 3.3
k-NN	18.6 ± 2.1	78 ± 3.3	85 ± 3
Single tree	19.2 ± 1.9	82 ± 3.2	80 ± 3.4
SVM	20.9 ± 2	75 ± 3.5	83 ± 3.5
LDA	50.1 ± 3.7	49 ± 24	51 ± 30

Table 4.5 Seven machines analyzing the Stroke-B data, with original data (top), and pre-balanced data (bottom). As in Table 4.4, the machines are comparable in their conclusions, apart from the LDA, which again fails for this kind of data

Machine	Error rate	Sensitivity	Specificity
RF	14.7 ± 1.5	85 ± 2.5	86 ± 2.1
k-NN	16.5 ± 1.8	84 ± 2.6	83 ± 2.6
NN	18.8 ± 1.7	79 ± 2.8	83 ± 2.6
Single tree	20.5 ± 1.6	80 ± 2.8	79 ± 2.7
Boosting	21.1 ± 1.7	75 ± 2.7	83 ± 2.6
SVM	22.2 ± 1.4	75 ± 2.8	81 ± 2.7
LDA	50.3 ± 7.4	51 ± 32	49 ± 46
RF	13.2 ± 1.3	86 ± 2.2	87 ± 2.3
NN	15.3 ± 1.5	84 ± 2.6	86 ± 2.3
Single tree	18.9 ± 1.8	81 ± 2.7	81 ± 3
k-NN	20.1 ± 8.4	80 ± 5.9	79 ± 22
Boosting	21.2 ± 1.9	76 ± 2.6	82 ± 2.8
SVM	21.9 ± 1.6	75 ± 3.4	82 ± 2.7
LDA	50.2 ± 6.3	42 ± 24	58 ± 27

Notes

(1) In this example we used three linear decision boundaries to separate the at-risk from normal subjects. Each of these boundaries was motivated by the clinical literature. However, our choice of the cut-points for each of these boundaries is only suggestive of the truly complicated biology of cardiac risk and its interactions with cholesterol, which itself occurs in several forms. That is: (a) we have excluded triglyceride levels from this discussion, and this is itself a critical part of evaluating health risk, as well as a standard part of calculating LDL from total cholesterol. In this simulated example, therefore, total cholesterol is just LDL+HDL. Also, properly including triglyceride would have led to a three-dimensional measurement space, and we chose a simpler sample space. (b) The lower limit for HDL is, from the literature, a possible symptom of entirely noncardiac problems. (c) Finally, the ratio limit of 4 for LDL/HDL also excludes the triglyceride value, as the correct numerator should be total cholesterol. We recommend taking the medical accuracy of these three boundaries with a massive grain of salt – which is certainly not good for cardiac health.

On the other hand, the cut-points and functions we used were in fact suggested using *another* learning machine: Google. This gateway to the Universe generates a short list from all sampled sites and induces a ranking among them. It is an example of an astonishingly successful, *unsupervised* learning machine; see the discussion in Chapter 3.

(2) In studying the performance of any algorithm, the method of using simulated, computer-generated data is sometimes called the *Monte Carlo* approach. We prefer using *simulated* for this method.

(3) A fuzzy boundary for the cholesterol data can be generated this way: (a) calculate the shortest distance, d, of a point to the boundary; (b) for that point assign the probability that the membership of the point implied by the boundary is *reversed* using an exponential decay function, $PV(\text{point at distance } d) = 0.5 \exp(-d/d_\tau)$; (c) in Figure 4.3(a) let $d_\tau = 5$. In words, away from the boundary the point is correctly assigned with increasing confidence to be at risk, not at risk, and on the boundary it is assigned at risk, not at risk with probability 0.5.

(4) It is desired generally that a labor-intensive, fine-tuning of a model should not be necessary. In applying a support vector machine we explored three different kernels – linear, cubic, and radial basis – and several values of the cost factor parameter. When the best possible selections and values are chosen it appears that the choice of a kernel is not very important and all three kernels yield similar error rates, as seen in Figure 4.7. However, in the case of linear and cubic kernels the error rate can reach 30% and 19%, respectively, for a different setting of the cost factor, while for the radial basis function it remains stable. When using more balanced data and without the fuzzy boundary this difference in performance across just these three kernels becomes even more drastic, from 2% to 35%. A good learning machine shouldn't be this hard to use.

Part II

A machine toolkit

Logistic regression

No, no, you're not thinking; you're just being logical.

Niels Bohr

5.1 Introduction

We introduce here the logistic regression model. It is a widely used statistical technique in biomedical data analysis, for a number of reasons.

First, it estimates the probability of a case belonging to a group – in principle this provides more information than simply deciding (yes, no) to which group a case belongs. Moreover, the probability estimates can be turned into predictions.

Second, it is fairly easy to interpret, as the (log odds of the) probability is expressed as a linear weighted sum of the features, much like a regression analysis.

Third, like regression analysis, the coefficients in the model can (with similar care) be interpreted as positive or negative associations of the variables with the predicted probability. For example, individual genes or clinical findings can be assigned protective or risk values expressed as log odds.

As will be discussed in Chapters 8 and 9, there are problems with interpreting any regression models, yet compared to the other statistical learning machines we eventually discuss, logistic regression is far easier to interpret. This is why we suggest first applying learning machines to the data, to identify the most informative features, then generating a simpler, equally accurate model – logistic regression – using just those features. The logistic regression model is an endpoint or reference model throughout this book.

We will not discuss in detail either the basic computational or advanced statistical aspects of logistic regression; see Note 1. Rather we will focus on how to use and interpret logistic regression, and identify some of its problems, including these five: (1) the consequences of defining an inter-action term in a model; (2) the distinction between estimating the probability of group membership and the simpler problem of making a yes/no predic-tion for belonging to a group; (3) the idea of using one model inside another; (4) obtaining a more practical, smaller and better-understood model, that is, logistic regression as a post-processing reference model; and (5) the problem of testing the goodness-of-fit for any logistic regression model, which turns out to be a formidable but solvable technical challenge.

Excellent general references for this topic include Harrell (2001), Hosmer and Lemeshow (2000), Hilbe (2009).

5.2 Inside and around the model

Consider tossing a single coin. We get *heads* with probability $\Pr(\text{heads}) = p$, and *tails* with probability $1 - p$. We repeatedly toss the coin, and assume that such tosses don't "see" each other – they are statistically independent. In a sequence of k tosses we find that:

$$\Pr(\text{number of heads is equal to } h) = \text{constant} \times p^h \times (1 - p)^{k-h} \quad (5.1)$$

(regarding the constant, see Note 2).

For convenience, we write:

$$\Pr(h; p, k) = \Pr(\text{number of heads is equal to } h \text{ after } k \text{ tosses}) \quad (5.2)$$

when the probability of a single head is equal to p, in k tosses. Note that in a sequence of k tosses, if we observe h heads, then we must necessarily observe $(k - h)$ tails. Thus the equation above fully states our probabilistic under-standing of the data, for which the (usually unknown) value p is the single parameter in this model.

Suppose now we start with a collection of two kinds of coins, some of which have a heads probability of p_1, others a heads probability of p_2. Assuming as before that the coin tosses are independent, we can first toss the p_1 coins a total of k_1 times, and then toss the p_2 coins a total of k_2 times. Under this simple tossing scheme we can write down a probability model for a sequence of $k = k_1 + k_2$ tosses. Suppose that we have observed h_1, h_2

heads in the two sets of tosses, for a total number of observed heads $h = h_1 + h_2$. Using the assumption of statistical independence for the full set of coin tosses, then standard probability tells us that

$$\text{Pr(total number of heads} = h = h_1 + h_2) = \text{Pr}(h_1; k_1, p_1) \times \text{Pr}(h_2; k_2, p_2). \tag{5.3}$$

Allowing the probability of observing a head on any single toss (the two values of p above) to vary across tosses is one way to slightly generalize the original coin-tossing experiment.

Here is another way: allow the heads probabilities, the ps, to be functions of other variables, for example type of coin, when it was tossed, where the tossing took place, etc. That is, we introduce the probability of heads as a function,

$$p = f(x_1, x_2, \ldots, x_m), \tag{5.4}$$

where the xs are measurements or grouping variables or, more generally, arbitrary features. In this expanded coin-tossing experiment the probability of heads changes over the many tosses, since each case has its associated list of features. As in Eq. (5.3) above, this leads to a final probability statement for the total number of heads that is a product over all the separate bits of probability. As we've just witnessed, models of this form can get quite complex very quickly, but in this teeming class there is a very useful, simple way to organize the model. The more mathematical details are given in Note 3.

5.3 Interpreting the coefficients

In a single logistic regression equation consider holding constant all the x measurements (features), save for a single one, say x_1. That is, we agree to statistically *condition* on all the other xs, the features $x_2, x_3, \ldots$. Then, when x_1 is increased by one unit, the log odds of the outcome (heads, say) is increased by a_1, which is the weight (coefficient) for this feature in the model. Similarly for all the other coefficients and unit measurement increases in those measurements, when everything else is held fixed; see Note 4.

5.4 Using logistic regression as a decision rule

A logistic regression model, one that generates probabilities, can be turned into a binary decision rule. Choose a threshold or cut-point, c, such that

$$\text{declared at risk if log odds} > c,$$
$$\text{declared normal if log odds} \leq c. \tag{5.5}$$

Now any decision rule incurs two kinds of error: declaring Group 2 for a case that correctly belongs to Group 1, and the reverse, declaring Group 1 for a case that correctly belongs to Group 2. We try to match or equalize the two kinds of error; see Chapter 11.

5.5 Logistic regression applied to the cholesterol data

We now apply two logistic regression models to the cholesterol data introduced in Chapter 4.

Begin by defining the model

$$\text{log odds} = a + b \times \text{HDL} + c \times \text{LDL}, \tag{5.6}$$

where a, b, and c are the coefficients that are estimated from the data.

We apply this model to the simulated cholesterol data, a single instance of which is displayed in Figure 4.1, and find that

$$\hat{a} = 0.087, \quad \hat{b} = -0.004, \quad \hat{c} = -14.123. \tag{5.7}$$

As a decision threshold we find a cut-point such that the two error values, at risk classified as normal, normal classified as at risk, are approximately equal. One cut-point, chosen to minimize *overall* error, is 0.198, so that:

$$\text{declared at risk if log odds} > 0.198,$$
$$\text{declared normal if log odds} \leq 0.198. \tag{5.8}$$

The decisions for these cases are displayed in Figure 5.1. As shown in the figure, the apparent error rates for this decision rule are not especially good, or, at least are confusing That is, equivalently, the sensitivity and specificity are quite unequal. This results in part from the basic unbalanced nature of the data; more precisely, it is not a deficiency of the logistic regression model

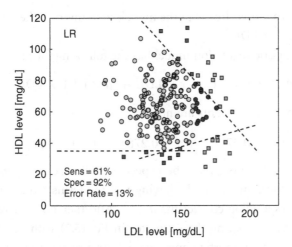

Figure 5.1   A logistic regression model was applied to the simulated cholesterol data. No interaction term was included, nor was any correction for unbalanced group sizes applied. The model performance is not especially good.

- at risk, misclassified as normal
- normal, correctly classified as normal
- normal, misclassified as at risk
- at risk, correctly classified as at risk

or the software used. See Chapter 12 for more on unbalanced data. One possible remedy for this inequality of error rate is to change the threshold (cut-point) that we use to define the decision rule. We give two examples of changing the threshold, below, for this same data.

These unequal accuracy measures, sensitivity and specificity, also might have been expected, along with the relatively high error rate, since any threshold value for this particular model amounts to deciding at risk vs. normal using *any* single line, where to one side of the line we decide *at risk*, and to the other side we decide *normal*. By inspection of the data in Figure 5.1, the normal group is not well modeled using a *single* above/below-the-line rule.

As an attempt to improve the model we now introduce an interaction term. In somewhat complex datasets such as this one an interaction term of some kind is often the automatic next step. However, the notion of interaction is mathematically and biologically not an easily framed idea; more on this in Chapter 9. Nonetheless, interaction is often understood to be simply the product of two terms already in the model, so in this case the interaction is defined as HDL × LDL.

The revised logistic regression model has the following form:

$$\log \text{odds} \ = \ a \ + \ b \times \text{HDL} \ + \ c \times \text{LDL} \ + \ d \times \text{HDL} \times \text{LDL}, \quad (5.10)$$

where the estimated coefficients are now:

$$\hat{a} = 40.9647, \quad \hat{b} = -0.9771, \quad \hat{c} = -0.2784, \quad \hat{d} = 0.0063. \quad (5.11)$$

The estimated coefficients should be expected to change, sometimes dramatically, from those in the model having just the terms {constant, HDL, LDL}, with corresponding coefficients a, b, c. And they do so here, as the reader can see by comparing the estimates in Eq. (5.7) with those in Eq. (5.11). To repeat this important message, how a predictor or variable or covariate operates in a given model is a function of all the other terms in the model; see Chapter 9.

Using a threshold of 0.13 (as in Eq. (5.8)), the decision region for this model with interaction is displayed in Figure 5.2. In this figure we have used a newly simulated batch of cholesterol data.

The estimated error rate for this model, 0.27, is a little over twice what we got for the model without interaction, 0.13.

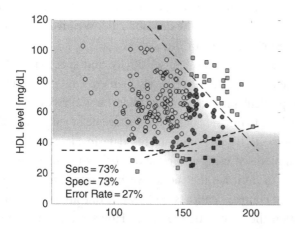

Figure 5.2   Logistic regression for simulated cholesterol data. This model has an interaction term and a threshold of 0.13, chosen to equalize the sensitivity and specificity.

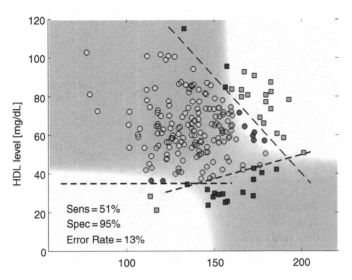

Figure 5.3   Logistic regression for simulated cholesterol data. This model has an interaction term and a threshold of 0.35, chosen to minimize the overall error.

Let's try and reduce the overall error by adjusting the threshold. See Figure 5.3 for this revised model, where a threshold of 0.35 was applied. Here we see that the error, 0.13, is back to what we got for the no-interaction model, but the other two performance measures, sensitivity and specificity, are very unequal. That is, we make an error of deciding at risk for some normal patients of about $1 - 0.95 = 0.05$ (which is good), but make the reverse error of deciding normal for many at-risk patients of about $1 - 0.51 = 0.49$ (which is very not good).

For the simulated cholesterol data in Figure 5.4 we used a threshold of 0.5. This would seem to make some sense as we are then choosing to declare a patient at risk if the estimated probability (using the model with interaction) is above 0.5, and declare a patient normal otherwise. However, the overall error does look good, 0.10, while we are also evidently coin-tossing (with probability = 0.5) in making a decision about the at risk patients, and declaring every normal patient to be not at risk. This makes sense, therefore, only if the cost of declaring a patient as normal when they are in fact at risk is essentially zero compared to declaring a patient as at risk when they are in fact normal. Such arguments require very careful assessments of misclassification costs, and prevalence of at-risk patients in the population under

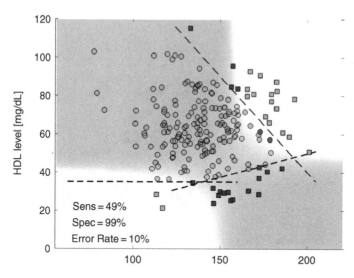

Figure 5.4   Logistic regression for simulated cholesterol data. This model has an interaction term and a threshold of 0.5.

- ▪ at risk, misclassified as normal
- ○ normal, correctly classified as normal
- ● normal, misclassified as at risk
- ▪ at risk, correctly classified as at risk

study. This leads to the still-developing subject of clinical decision theory; see Hilden (2004).

However, there is another problem revealed in all three figures, Figures 5.2, 5.3, and 5.4. The decision boundaries for each are areas marked off by the two shaded regions of unusual shape. Let's consider how these decision boundaries arose.

5.6 A cautionary note

The decision boundary in the example above is defined, as a mathematical object, by two hyperbolas. For this reason the threshold rule for the model leads to the anomalous prediction in the shaded lower right corners of each of Figures 5.2, 5.3, and 5.4, where definitely at-risk patients have been misclassified as normal. That is, using this very frequently used form for the interaction, the multiplicative term HDL × LDL leads to an unexpected decision boundary: the two sections mapped out by a *pair* of hyperbolas. In fact, any new case appearing in the lower right shaded region would be misclassified as normal, no matter how far it was from the majority of the normal cases. Such cases might be infrequent, as was true in our simulation, but this is a worrisome feature of a model with interaction. We could repair this boundary with more care in choosing one "branch" of the hyperbola. Surely some repair of the model is demanded, as no clinician would be expected to endorse a prediction method that makes such profound errors so systematically.

The more important point here is that automatic and often unthinking use of a multiplicative interaction term can have unintended and certainly unwanted consequences. And the problem is not limited to logistic regression models, nor to multiplicative interaction terms. That is, decision rules can be quite complex in problems with many more predictors and many more dimensions in which these hyperbolic (or other complex) decision boundaries are being introduced. Hence even if it were the case that "interaction" should be defined as the product of two features, it is not clear in higher-dimension problems (with many more features) if we can always mathematically repair the boundaries using some branch-selection scheme within the logistic regression framework. Such a method would delete the lower right shaded region in Figure 5.2, for example, but how do we monitor such shaded regions in higher dimensions and eliminate just the spurious ones?

Let's push a little harder and look at the consequences of the hyperbola decision boundaries in a model with interaction. Our comments here don't apply to just logistic regression problems.

Suppose it is true that by working a little harder we can get the upper left hyperbola region to very nicely comport with the normal subjects in the data. Or, simply suppose that randomly the data for the normal subjects, and only the normals, fit into the upper left hyperbola given by the logistic regression. That is, we find an upper left hyperbola that doesn't misclassify any normal subject and also doesn't step over any line and misclassify an at-risk case as normal. The lower right hyperbola might then include more or fewer at-risk subjects, and would declare all of them, incorrectly, as normal. Suppose further, that the data we collect has, again randomly, no subjects in the general area of the lower right hyperbola. This section of the decision rule would then be making no mistakes, which is presumably a good thing.

Indeed, in this case the decision rule given by the two branches of the hyperbola would make no mistakes on the training data.

There are two curious facets of this apparently good result, one mathematically interesting but without other consequence, the other data-dependent and very consequential.

First, we've been talking about optimally adjusted branches of *hyperbolas* but it is also true that with this very nice, if somewhat complex interaction model, we're back to a linear model. Here is what is going on. The logistic model is using three features, LDL, HDL, and a product term LDL × HDL. As far as the computer code for this method, or the final prediction itself, is concerned, the product term could be written MULT = LDL × HDL, and then the decision scheme for the model takes this form:

Let $y = a + b \times \text{LDL} + c \times \text{HDL} + d \times \text{MULT}$;

Choose normal if $y \leq C$, and at risk if $y > C$

(where we choose the constant C in some optimal way). Expressed this way, the decision rule is linear in the features {LDL, HDL, MULT}, and all subjects on one side of this plane (in this feature space of three dimensions) are classified as normal, and those on the other side are classified as at risk. The model is not linear in the original data, which is simply the pair of measurements {LDL, HDL}.

Second, the model is successfully making decisions using a linear function, and as long as there (randomly) happen to be no at-risk subjects in the lower branch of the hyperbola pair, and no normals outside the upper branch, the training data is said to be linearly separable. For the logistic regression model the coefficients cannot be derived, and this is a well-known hazard of any logistic model. For the more technically inclined, the likelihood function for estimating the model parameters has no finite maximum and the code doesn't converge. This curious event can arise with just two data points; see the discussion of maximum likelihood estimation in Freedman (2009, p. 149). The ability of straight lines or planes to separate random finite sets of points is related to the *VC* dimension of the family of purely linear methods; see DGL (chapter 13; especially corollary 13.1).

The conclusion is that the training data, in having no at-risk subjects in the far lower right of Figure 5.3, suggests that a pair of hyperbolas can be very good decision boundaries, but this excellent decision scheme is *inaccessible* using standard logistic regression. Deleting training data points won't help here; collecting more data might. Even a single normal subject out of place, say appearing in the lower right region, would yield data that is no longer linearly separable.

Including interactions or any higher-order terms in any model can lead us far astray. And not all unintended consequences of mathematically more sophisticated models can even be easily located, let alone repaired. More optimistically, see Zhao and Liu (2007).

5.7 Another cautionary note

When used with care, logistic regression can be a very useful tool. One caution, also valid in classical linear regression, is that the features often have significantly unequal variances, so increasing a feature by "one unit" (while holding fixed the values for all the other features) should not be expected to have the same change in outcome as increasing another feature. A standard method for dealing with this complication is to transform all the features to new ones with (at least approximately) unit variance. However, while it puts each feature on a more equal footing in terms of ease of interpretation, it won't change the *correlation* structure of the predictors; see Note 5.

Also, just as changing variances for a feature in a decision tree will shift the cut-point for that feature at a node in the tree, the changed variances in a logistic regression will shift the coefficient of a feature up or down. More generally, while standardizing the feature variances will change the appearance of some aspects of a model, it won't change the accuracy of the prediction being made, or the probability estimate, when the machine is rerun using the standardized features.

Certain mathematical and computational problems are also inherent in logistic regression. For example, if it is true that the two groups, survived or not survived, can be completely separated in a geometrical sense (the groups have a separating hyperplane in the space of features), then the usual estimation scheme (maximum likelihood) provably never converges. This is peculiar, of course, since if the groups are so cleanly defined in terms of the measurements, then we might expect estimation to be trivial and most certainly not explode.

Another problem is closely related to the one just discussed. The model coefficients cannot easily be obtained when the features $x = \{x_1, x_2, \ldots, x_r\}$

always, or mostly, satisfy a linear relationship or constraint. In this case the data, x, lies entirely *on* a hyperplane. An example: the measurements are proportions, so that

$$x_1 + x_2 + \ldots + x_r = 1. \tag{5.14}$$

In either of these troublesome cases, sensible software will warn us that convergence was not possible. Then we must consider alternatives, such as: use fewer measurements, define new covariates based on the old ones, or use an entirely different learning machine method.

These solutions are not without their own sets of problems. For example, if we choose to drop a feature simply because it is correlated with other features, then we might be tossing out a quite useful feature. To avoid such dilemmas, we suggest avoiding this selection process of removing features, and instead recommend relying on a statistical learning machine to do good variable selection for us. Again, part of our modeling strategy is to use learning machines for the heavy lifting, as it were, and then engineer a return to more familiar, smaller models, such as linear or logistic regression.

5.8 Probability estimates and decision rules

The logistic regression model takes measurement values and returns a value of the log odds ratio for each subject. Assuming the model is accurate, the estimated probability outcome for each subject may be more informative than a simple declaration of each subject being in one group or the other, but this reuse of the model is context-dependent; see Harrell (2001, section 10.8). In sorting out the question of whether to seek a decision rule or probability estimate for each subject, we advance our understanding of how a logistic regression model operates, and how we might expect any statistical learning machine to behave. See also Note 6 in Chapter 2, for more background on this subject.

Consider the fact that a subject far from a proposed decision boundary may not be very useful by itself for estimating the boundary. For a decision problem we are interested in skillfully locating (statistically estimating) the boundary itself, so that subjects clearly far from the boundary are *possibly* irrelevant to the decision process. That is, *if* we think that the decision problem is the main research issue, it only matters if the boundary is efficiently located.

On the other hand, using a decision cut-point for a logistic regression model undermines the usefulness of reporting a probability for a given subject. Different estimated probabilities for different subjects could lead to alternative diagnostic pathways, or identification of important subsets in the data. *If* the probability estimates are valid then reducing a logistic regression to just a decision rule is wasteful.

As a practical matter, it can be hard to validate a cut-point decision rule that is originally based on a logistic regression model for the probability of group membership. How should we efficiently compare estimated probabilities derived from equally plausible but distinct models? This is a nontrivial question and there is a correspondingly huge literature on evaluation of diagnostic and predictive models; see Zhou *et al.* (2002), Hand (1997), Pepe (2003). These sources emphasize the technique of *receiver operator curves* (ROC plots) to interrogate the output of any decision rule based on a cut-point.

Other rigorous treatments of this problem place it in the context of *proper scoring* rules. Here the goal is to weight probability estimates – such as are provided by a logistic regression model – by the estimated costs of incorrect estimates; see Predd *et al.* (2009). Under this assessment, ROC plots are not deemed satisfactory as analytic tools for evaluating probability estimates, as they are easily shown to be *improper* scoring rules

Summarizing so far, an estimated probability of group membership for a subject will be generically more informative that simply a binary decision for the subject, but *simply* making {yes, no} decisions is often exactly the problem at hand.

5.9 Evaluating the goodness-of-fit of a logistic regression model

There exists a family of methods for evaluating a logistic regression's probability estimates. Using the stroke data we apply a SAS macro, %GOFLOGIT, developed by Oliver Kuss, which generates many of the current crop of global measures for testing the goodness-of-fit of any logistic regression model; see Kuss (2002), Hu *et al.* (2006).

We begin by generating a model using the Stroke-A data, with 38 of the available features. There are $N = 1114$ subjects, with 557 complete restitution and 557 incomplete or partial restitution subjects. The data is sufficiently complex that no subject has the same values for all 38 features as any other subject. Such data in the logistic regression community is called *sparse*. This poses a problem for probability estimation *if* probability estimation is the basis for evaluating the goodness-of-fit of the model. That is, we can't easily pool subjects together to get some sense of their common, true probability of group membership, given that each subject is fully distinct from every other: a probability estimate is not easily constructed with a single data point (that is, the list of the values of the features for that subject).

Sparse data means that some of the standard tests for the goodness-of-fit of a logistic model simply breakdown altogether. Under complete sparsity, the measure called residual deviance, D, becomes a statistic that is completely independent of the observations and hence contains no information about the model fit; see Kuss (2002, p. 3791). In addition, the Pearson statistic is, under complete sparsity, approximately equal to the sample size, so it too is not a sensible measure of fit; see Kuss (2002, p. 3792). Continuing with this litany of collapse, the Farrington statistic reduces to exactly the sample size. Finally, the very widely used Hosmer–Lemeshow test under sparsity yields p-values that are highly unstable. Kuss (2002) considers other problems with this familiar procedure.

In a much more positive direction there are many other procedures that do well, with sparse or not-sparse data, and are to be recommended. These are: RSS, IM, and the statistics developed by Osius and McCullagh; see Kuss (2002) for details. We now apply all these methods, good or not so good, to the Stroke-A data.

In Table 5.1 the *number of unique profiles* is the number of groups of subjects that are distinguishable in terms of their features. With 1114 such unique profiles, the data is by definition maximally sparse. The deviance statistic, more correctly the residual deviance, can be shown, under sparseness, to be independent of the outcomes for each subject. The Pearson statistic is 1222.0534, that is, basically the size of the sample, 1114. The null hypothesis for each test is that the logistic model does fit the data. But observe that the p-value for the residual deviance will essentially never reject a model, under sparseness, as it's always too large, while the Pearson statistic is at the other extreme and will nearly always reject the null, as it's always too small. Neither test is helpful for sparse data. The Farrington test (not displayed in Table 5.1) is also in this category. Its value for the stroke data is exactly zero, with a p-value of exactly 1.000.

Moving on to the actually useful goodness-of-fit statistics we find in Table 5.2: again, the null hypothesis for all tests is that the logistic regression model having 38 features fits the Stroke-A data, so that the non-significance of these four tests allows us to not reject the null.

Finally, there is a slightly different line of thinking about goodness-of-fit tests for the logistic model, given in Hu *et al.* (2006). They argue that the test statistic, R^2, familiar from ordinary linear regression *can* be used for logistic modeling, provided that the model is correct and that large sample theory is applied. That is, R^2 in large samples does approximate the explained variation in the model much as it does in the linear regression context. They also discuss another test statistic not considered by Kuss (2002), the Gini

Table 5.1 Two classical methods, Pearson correlation and deviance, for evaluating the goodness-of-fit for a logistic regression model as applied to Stroke A. For the given data neither one is appropriate, as the data is completely sparse: the number of unique profiles exactly equals the sample size

Criterion	Value	DF	Value/DF	Pr > ChiSq
Deviance	981.2186	1075	0.9128	0.9808
Pearson	1222.0534	1075	1.1368	0.0011

Number of unique profiles: 1114.

Table 5.2 The result of applying four alternative methods for evaluating the goodness-of-fit for a logistic regression model as applied to Stroke A. These methods are provably good for sparse data; technical details are given in Kuss (2002). In all four tests, the null hypothesis is that the given model does fit the data. Since all p-values are nonsignificant here, we choose to accept the null hypothesis

Statistic	Value	p-Value
Osius test	1.124	0.131
McCullagh test	1.092	0.137
IM test	46.000	0.205
RSS test	159.014	0.484

concentration measure, but find that it is problematic for several technical and practical reasons; see Note 5.

The focus in Hu *et al.* (2006) is on trying to recover the linear regression *idea* of R^2, that is, as a statistic for seeing how well the variation in the data is "explained" by the model. Kuss and others (personal communication) correctly point out that a goodness-of-fit statistic measures the difference between observed and fitted values, and so is conceptually distinct from a statistic that generates an *explanation* of variation. This is a nontrivial distinction. On the other hand, we think both points of view are helpful in the study of logistic regression models.

5.10 Calibrating a logistic regression

We have noted above that a logistic regression model can generate a single value for every subject, specifically the log odds for that subject. From this we can calculate the probability of class membership for that subject. As in Section 5.9, suppose our interest is in using this estimated probability and we would like to evaluate the estimate, that is, see how good it is at estimating the true probability of group membership for a given subject.

Usually we don't have a competing estimate of the membership of group probability that could be considered a gold standard. So simply collecting more data or using a test dataset is not exactly an answer here. The problem is that for each subject we are not, under logistic regression, estimating a quantity that can be directly observed and then confirmed or validated. The probability of an occurrence for a specific subject is not measured as, say, total cholesterol for the subject.

Nonetheless, we can generate *competing* estimated probabilities for all the subjects in the data, and see if the estimates are in approximate agreement. One method for doing so was introduced by Cox (1958). See also Harrell (2001, section 10.9) and Note 6. A real-world example of calibrating a logistic regression model, using the stroke data discussed in Chapter 4, is given in König *et al.* (2008). The calibration idea can be generalized in several ways for a wide range of learning machines, as we discuss below.

Here is the method: given a logistic regression (or other) model we proceed to use that model as a *single* new "feature" to be used in training another logistic regression on the test data. This may seem circular and not likely to be very informative, but consider how the old model might appear in, be part of, the new model. That is, if the original model appears unmodified and unadjusted – *unrefined* – as a useful predictor in the new model, then it is reasonable to conclude that the original model is a good one. If the original model appears with some adjustment (some nonzero coefficient in the new model) then presumably the original model benefits from this calibration step. More precisely, for both the original model and the new one (generated on the test data) we can compare the case probability estimates given by these two logistic regression models on the new data. In this way we can plot the probabilities estimated by the original model against those estimated by using the new model, where the single predictor is the probability estimate of the old model.

There are a number of assumptions and caveats required to be considered: (a) both models, old and new, are good fits to both sets of data; (b) the two datasets are drawn from the single population of interest; (c) our intent is to refine or improve the original model; (d) refining the original model here is definitely *not* the same as validating the model, and refinement here means studying the stability of the original model under the challenge of new data.

Depending on the amount of modification, adjustment, or more precisely the amount of calibration required to adapt the old model in light of the new data, we could go on to improve the original model; see Note 7.

We use the cholesterol data to see how calibration works, and begin by generating (simulating) new datasets in two ways. The first method does this: generate a dataset, fit a logistic regression (LR) model, LR(1), and then generate many additional replicates of the original data. On each of these second datasets we fit another logistic regression model, LR(2), of an especially simple type: LR(1) is used as input, a single feature, for the second logistic regression model, LR(2). For example, one version of LR(2) has the form:

$$LR(2) = \log \text{odds} = e + f \times LR(1), \tag{5.20}$$

where

$$LR(1) = \log \text{odds} = \hat{a} + \hat{b} \times HDL + \hat{c} \times LDL + \hat{d} \times HDL \times LDL, \tag{5.21}$$

for

$$\hat{a} = -0.1154, \quad \hat{b} = -0.6103, \quad \hat{c} = 0.0039, \quad \hat{d} = 17.0703. \qquad (5.22)$$

The idea is that if LR(1) is a stable model, then the estimate for e in Eq. (5.20) should be approximately zero, *and* the estimate for f in Eq. (5.20) should be approximately one. Such an estimation result states that LR(1) needs no appreciable adjustment when applied to new data. Any adjustment we derive would serve to *calibrate* the logistic modeling process, leading to a revised version of the original model.

As noted above, it is essential to recognize that (a) this revision is not a new model, with other features incorporated, others deleted; and (b) this calibration step does not yield a validation of the model in the sense that the probability estimates for each subject are somehow being improved.

To simulate the consequences of logistic calibration, we first generated 3×100 additional versions of the data: data(1) and data(2). That is, three versions (Runs 1, 2, and 3) of the original data, = data(1), were generated each with 500 data points, and then 100 versions of additional data, = data (2), were generated. For each pair of datasets {data(1), data(2)} a model of the form LR(1) was estimated using data(1), and then that was used as input to a model LR(2) for data(2). For these three runs, the following mean values, standard errors, and 95% confidence intervals for e and f were obtained:

$$
\begin{array}{lll}
f: & 1.0053 \pm 0.168085 & (\text{SE } 0.000532) \\
e: & 0.0084 \pm 0.210013 & (\text{SE } 0.000664)
\end{array}
$$

$$
\begin{array}{lll}
f: & 1.0867 \pm 0.212531 & (\text{SE } 0.000672) \\
e: & 0.1966 \pm 0.239148 & (\text{SE } 0.000756)
\end{array} \qquad (5.23)
$$

$$
\begin{array}{lll}
f: & 1.1354 \pm 0.152095 & (\text{SE } 0.000481) \\
e: & 0.0892 \pm 0.202352 & (\text{SE } 0.000640).
\end{array}
$$

The six 95% z-score confidence intervals for *each* of these six terms – the *e*s and the *f*s – do *not* contain 1.0 or zero, for each *f* or *e*, respectively. Note that in these six intervals above we used simulations over many runs to get the means and standard errors, while in a single run of a logistic regression program these intervals are standard output (or, at least, the standard errors for the slope and intercept are routinely given).

Hence each of these three runs points to the presence of bias in the LR(1) model based on data(2), and calibration is suggested. Note that all three runs suggest the same direction for the corresponding adjustments, so that the four uncalibrated coefficients in LR(1) need two adjustments, one to greatly lower the intercept term, a, and another to slightly raise the regression terms, b, c, and d.

The standard interpretation of the required re-estimations for the four model terms goes this way:

(a) if $e > 0$ then the predicted log odds using LR(1) are too low, and are too high if $e > 0$;
(b) if $|f| > 1$ then the regression terms b, c, d in LR(1) need to be increased, as they are said to be not sufficiently varying;
(c) if $0 < |f| < 1$ then the original regression terms vary too much;
(d) if $f > 0$ then the regression terms are all at least in the right direction;
(e) if $f < 0$ then the regression terms are in the wrong direction.

Furthermore, adjustments to the intercept in the LR(1) model, through the e coefficient are more strictly said to be *calibration*, while adjustments to the regression terms, through the f coefficient are said to be *refinements* to the original LR(1) model; see Miller *et al.* (1993).

We can declare the LR(2) model, using the es and fs, to be the adjusted or calibrated model, or, we can refer back to the original model LR(1) and make the suggested adjustment:

$$\text{LR(1)}_{\text{adjusted}} = \hat{a}_{\text{adj}} + \hat{b}_{\text{adj}} \times \text{HDL} + \hat{c}_{\text{adj}} \times \text{LDL} + \hat{d}_{\text{adj}} \times \text{HDL} \times \text{LDL}$$

(5.24)

where using the first pair of estimates for e and f in Eq. (5.23) we find:

$$\hat{a}_{\text{adj}} = (0.0084) \times (-0.1154) = -0.00097,$$
$$\hat{b}_{\text{adj}} = (1.0053) \times (-0.6103) = -0.61353,$$
$$\hat{c}_{\text{adj}} = (1.0053) \times (0.0039) = 0.00392,$$
$$\hat{d}_{\text{adj}} = (1.0053) \times (17.0703) = 17.16077.$$

(5.25)

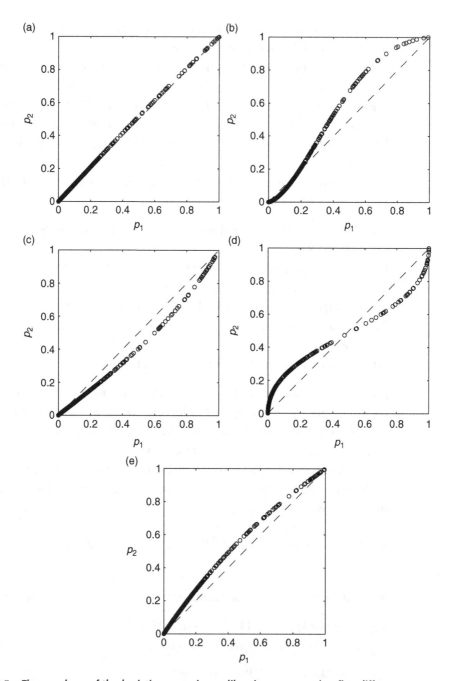

Figure 5.5   Five versions of the logistic regression calibration curve, using five different simulations of the cholesterol data.

Here is another version of the calibration process using a different simulation scheme. We generated an initial dataset, data(1), and then generated another dataset, data(2). Each pair {data(1), data(2)} was therefore generated 100 times. This led to:

$$f: \quad 0.9676 \pm 0.2191 \quad (\text{SE } 0.000693)$$
$$e: \quad -0.0233 \pm 0.2809 \quad (\text{SE } 0.000888). \tag{5.26}$$

Once again, the z-score 95% confidence intervals for f and e suggest that bias is present in the LR(1) model, as the intervals don't contain 1 or 0, respectively. But now the uncalibrated estimates for the four model terms are apparently too low *or* too high. Thus, whatever adjustment we might make using the previous three runs are opposite to those we might now make. This instability suggests that the logistic regression model is probably not fitting the original data very well.

Furthermore, the plot of the estimated probabilities for *another* five instances of this process appear in Figure 5.5, where p_1 is the estimated probability for each subject in data(2) using LR(1) and p_2 is that for the same subject using LR(2). It is seen that LR(1) both over- and under-estimates the case probabilities, relative to the subject's probabilities derived using LR(2).

5.11 Beyond calibration

Our discussion of calibrating a logistic regression model is entangled with a number of other important ideas and each requires comment.

The plots above assume that the p_2 values as determined from LR(2) are close to the true probabilities for each subject, when in fact these values are themselves estimates for each case using the additional data. Any calibration using the p_2 values as "truth" is therefore somewhat misleading, so calibration in this sense means only an adjustment using a new set of estimated probabilities for each subject. This leads to the question, why not use the "new" data in some combination with the original "old" data to derive a single LR model based on twice the sample size. For example, resampling methods (Chapter 10) instead strive to pull all the available data together, old and new, training and test, into a single averaged model.

The error values for all these LR models, on any of data(1) or data(2), are all rather high, certainly when compared to the single decision tree approach, as we saw in Chapter 4. Hence it might not make practical sense to try calibrating any of these LR models for this data as above, instead of simply using a different model entirely. Otherwise expressed, when some significant calibration seems called for, or, if the calibration seems unstable as we noticed above, then we should look for alternative models.

Looking carefully at the results above, where we generated a *single* version of data(1) and then many versions of data(2), we find that the single data calibration method produced estimates for e and f that had lower standard errors, when compared to those cases where many versions of data(1) and data(2) were used. This is an important issue, in fact, for model building generally: when studying the accuracy of any modeling scheme, there is an inherent variability in the model generation itself. It is not, therefore, usually sufficient to generate a single model from the data and then test it on replicates. One must also consider both sources of variation, that for *generating* a model and that for *testing* it. Important attention has been given to this problem in the literature, but it seems to have only infrequently been acknowledged; see especially Molinaro *et al.* (2005). Some statistical learning machine methods take this into account automatically (Random Forests and Random Jungles), and some do not, at least in their native versions. However, the user can, with modest additional programming, set up bootstrap, cross-validation, and other resampling schemes.

It might be more systematic to include a calibration step as part of the original model generation process. Options for doing this include penalized maximum likelihood and shrinkage methods; see Moons *et al.* (2004).

The calibration idea is not obviously limited to improving logistic regression models, and in principle could be considered for any statistical learning method. Indeed, the reuse of one model as a *feature* in another model is a strategy that can often alter the accuracy of the final model, where it might improve the accuracy or lower it. If we consider the summary scores in the lupus dataset analyzed in Chapter 4, Charlson and SEL Comorbidity, then using them as input to another classifier such as Random Forests can be thought of as making a calibration step for those features. But we also saw there that including them as features *along* with the individual features on which they were based, resulted in higher error values when Random Forests was applied. There, the summary scores each could outperform the separate raw scores, but when they were excluded the raw scores found the local decision boundary more accurately, when present in a multiple tree-building process, such as Random Forests.

Continuing with the idea of using the output from one machine as the input to another, in this more flexible approach there is no requirement to keep the same model (or machine) form, for example, as we did above in fitting one LR model inside another LR model. Indeed, one LR model can appear as a feature in a decision tree model, and conversely. This is probably one of the most important ideas we can retain from the calibration experience, that of using one model or one learning machine, inside another; see Note 7.

There is, finally, another issue related to calibration: we have assumed the form of the model, as given in LR(1) with or without an interaction term, does indeed fit the data. In the absence of other confirming evidence, this assumption is only that: a working premise. The problem is that it can be difficult to get unbiased estimates of the probability (or log odds) of group membership. On the other hand, declaring a procedure to be good as a pure decision or classification rule is usually much easier. Technically the distinction here is that estimating a probability of group membership requires estimating a continuous quantity, while declaring membership is binary, a zero–one process. For the binary decision, as reviewed in Chapter 2, we only need to come out on the correct side of the decision boundary, rather than estimating how far we are from the boundary.

5.12 Logistic regression and reference models

We now discuss the idea of a statistical reference model, at least for the problem of making classifications. We argue that a good model should:

(1) be simple, or *sparse*, involving just a handful of predictors or features, possibly including a short list of transformed or user-constructed features;
(2) exhibit good statistical properties, with acceptably low error values;
(3) enable relatively straightforward interpretation for the biomedical researcher;

(4) encourage relatively straightforward hypothesis generation, especially for designing the next experiment.

These criteria are jointly unattainable except in very special circumstances. However the criteria do provide guidance, in that if a prediction model is seriously deficient in any of these directions, then we would argue that our search for a good model is unfinished, at least for the given dataset and that biomedical problem.

For example, a model with a terrific accuracy rate (and balanced high sensitivity and specificity) might not be considered useful in itself if it required 100 features to be evaluated for every case, where many of the measurements came with high acquisition costs or inherent measurement inaccuracy. Also, an accurate but difficult to interpret model, one for which the user is uncertain as to the computer science or mathematics behind the decision-making process, would often not be adopted by the biomedical community. Validation is thus distinct from implementation and usage.

Closely related to this, is the fact that the bench scientist would be uncertain as to what experiments to pursue next, if the good accuracy resulted from using at least 1000 experimental variables (or genes, or SNPs) and not any fewer.

Or, adoption would be in doubt if the bench scientist approvingly noted the satisfyingly low error rate but could imagine no plausible explanation for the group separation as shown by the learning machine. In the absence of a plausible explanation the scientist is not provided with any path by which to explore the model, its implied biological pathways and contingencies. In the wider scientific drive to discover, it is probable that the model will simply be ignored.

It is also true, of course, that any classical linear model may still leave the user with nontrivial interpretation problems, even when the number of features in the model is quite small.

Given these limitations of any collection of attributes for a good model, what we will call a reference model for predictions, we still prefer to make an imperfect choice, and select the logistic regression model for this purpose. We do not insist that the logistic regression model is the *initial* model applied to our data. In our experience, especially with data having large numbers of features (anything more than 10, say) we strongly encourage the reader to apply learning machine methods first and then work back to simpler models, such as a logistic regression. Logistic regression and other more classical, parametric models are essential but often work best after the machine has done the heavy lifting of detecting signal in the data.

Notes

(1) For its depth and completeness we especially recommend Harrell (2001); see also the now-classic text by Hosmer and Lemeshow (2000, Second Edition). Excellent recent summaries of the benefits and hazards of logistic regression modeling can also be found in Ottenbacher *et al.* (2001, 2004). The emphasis in these sources is on small, parametric models. They don't discuss how logistic regression might fit into a machine learning approach to data analysis and they don't enter into a discussion of estimating group probability membership as might be conducted using statistical learning machines. As discussed in Section 5.9, Kuss (2002) and Hu *et al.* (2006) provide considerable detail and recent insight on logistic regression models.

(2) Here the constant $= k!/[(k-h)!h!] =$ the binomial coefficient. We use the mathematical notation

$$k! = k \cdot (k-1) \cdot (k-2) \cdot (k-3) \ldots (2)(1),$$

so for example, $5! = 5 \times 4 \times 3 \times 2 \times 1 = 120$.

(3) The features in a logistic regression model are not required to be multivariate normal as is the case with linear discriminant models, nor need they have *any* specific correlation or distributional structure. In this sense, a logistic model is distribution-free, but is still a parametric model, since we're estimating coefficients, one for each term in the model. Here is a logistic model with two parameters, *a* and *b*: log $[p/1-p] = a + bx$, where x is a feature, p is the probability of {survive} say, and the log term is the *log odds* of survival.

(4) Another issue with the process of conditioning on a set of features, to explore the consequences of changes in another feature, is that while it makes good mathematical sense to invoke conditioning to pursue this exploration, it is not clear that it always makes good biomedical or clinical sense. The problem is that for a given subject we are not necessarily free to move the value of a single feature up or down and

simply ignore the connection that feature has with all the others. The correlation structure of the data does not freely license this, unless the feature under study is statistically independent of all the others. This might be true, for instance, for input dials being set by the workers or researchers in a petrochemical processing plant. It might also be true for measurements obtained on subjects in a strictly controlled clinical trial, where subgroups of subjects are *assigned* diets, drugs, exercise regimens, etc. under monitoring. Changing a single feature in such models amounts to considering how patients might do *if* they had been in another arm of the trial, or under another clinical protocol following the analysis of the clinical trail. But for a single subject in an observational study, reasoning from this statistical conditioning is still problematic. The distinction here is between intervention and observation.

This convention concerning feature independence is often sadly underscored by an explicit assumption in some data analyses that the features in the logistic regression model must be statistically independent, or, at least uncorrelated with each other. This is a basic statistical mistake. It can lead to diminishing the perceived flexibility of logistic regression and then require a wholly unnecessary forced march in search of some alternative model. A marvelous discussion of observation, intervention, and much more, can be found in Freedman (2009) (see especially chapter 6).

(5) There is a detail here concerning variances of individual features that bears inspection. Some machines have the capacity to compare the predictive power of one feature against another. The two Randoms – Random Forests and Random Jungles – are good examples of such engines. It is known that if a feature has a high variance then a variable importance measure might more selectively choose that feature for inclusion in the model, thus raising its relative importance. The Gini method for calculating variable importances in Random Forests has this property; see Chapter 7. Unfortunately, this preference can lead to distorted or even incorrect feature rankings. See Strobl *et al.* (2007, 2008, 2009) and Nicodemus *et al.* (2009, 2010) for a discussion of the problem and suggested correctives.

Note as well that the problem Hu *et al.* (2006) found with use of the Gini concentration measure for evaluating the goodness-of-fit for a logistic regression model has a parallel with the important problem raised by Strobl *et al.* (2007, 2008). The Gini concentration appears to have an estimated large sample variance that is too small, and thus can seriously overstate the accuracy of the model when the specified model is not the correct one. Translation: the Gini value is more likely to pick the wrong model.

Finally, for some machines we are not required to rerun the data after standardizing the features. Indeed, some machines, such as statistically equivalent blocks, see only the so-called empirical distributions of the features, and so by design are scale-invariant; see DGL (section 11.4 and chapters 21, 22).

(6) The technique of calibration is closely related to that of shrinkage and penalized regression, as discussed for example in Steyerberg *et al.* (2004).

(7) This process of using one model inside another is related to the concept of *stacking*, as given in the regression context; see Wolpert (1992), Wolpert and Macready (1996), Übeyli (2006). There are important and deep mathematical results showing how to most efficiently stack, or more generally combine, any collection of models or machines of any type. See DGL (chapter 30) for the discussion of committee machines and how they relate to neural network machines. Generally, ensemble or committee methods work well when there is any signal in the data and the individual members of the committee are better than coin-tossing. In principle, given *any* set of prediction engines it can be shown that there is a kind of pooling method that is at least as good as the best method in the set, and indeed if one member of the set is Bayes optimal, then the combined method is also. For details, see Mojirsheibani (1999, 2002) and the discussion in Chapter 12. This is a remarkable, often easy to apply scheme, and deserves much more attention in both the statistical and the machine learning community.

A single decision tree

I never saw a discontented tree. They grip the ground as though they liked it, and though fast rooted they travel about as far as we do.

John Muir

6.1 Introduction

A method for making decisions that is both primitive and surprisingly effective is the *single decision tree*. It has a sound mathematical basis showing how well it does with large enough samples, and its extreme simplicity has led to a wide range of practical and effective variants. And generating many single trees lies at the heart of the Random Forests and Random Jungles procedures, which have been applied with increasing regularity and satisfying results.

Many good texts are available for decision trees, including Breiman *et al.* (1993), Hastie *et al.* (2009), Berk (2008). Mastering the details of tree growth and management is an excellent way to understand the activities of learning machines generally.

Let's begin our tree discussion with something near the end of the story: given a single tree, how does it make a decision?

6.2 Dropping down trees

Consider Figure 6.1. This is a single decision tree, derived using the at-risk boundaries we started with in Chapter 4. Let's assume for the moment that these at-risk determinations were constructed from the data, and that the three boundary lines in this example were estimated from the data. Now, for making predictions on a new subject the tree would work this way.

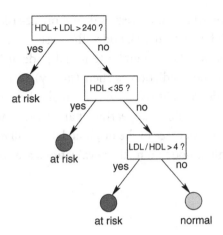

Figure 6.1   The decision tree for the simulated cholesterol data.

The values of each feature, for each subject, are examined in some order and the subject is dropped down the tree:

(1) At the top of Figure 6.1 the value for Feature 1, in this case the sum HDL + LDL, is examined first. The subject is moved down to the left if the sum is more than 240, and to the right if the sum is less than 240. That is, if HDL + LDL is less than 240 then the subject lands in a transition node (open box), or terminal node (dark gray circle) if at risk using this single function HDL + LDL.

(2) This splitting and sorting process continues. If the subject's HDL < 35 the subject is sent to the next terminal node (shaded dark gray). If HDL ≥ 35 the subject is dropped down to another transition node (another open box).

(3) One more check of the subject's values now occurs. If the ratio HDL/LDL is > 4 then the subject is sent to another terminal node, and if the ratio is ≤ 4 the subject is sent to the final terminal node (light gray circle).

Under this scheme every subject ultimately is dropped down to a terminal node, by definition one that is not split again. Note that we have yet to make a prediction for any subject, and only moved that person down the tree. The prediction step occurs this way. At each of the terminal nodes the proportion of at-risk compared to normal subjects is calculated, and a majority vote is taken in each node. That node will be an at-risk node if more at-risk subjects appear in that node, and will be a not-at-risk node otherwise. A new subject will eventually be dropped down the tree into a terminal node, using steps (1), (2), and (3) above, and the prediction is then (finally) simple: every subject at an at-risk node is declared at risk, and is normal otherwise.

Note especially that *every* new subject appearing at an at-risk node – one having a simple majority of at-risk cases in the original data – will *always* be declared at risk. At any terminal node no further evaluations are conducted for each new subject.

6.3 Growing a tree

The growth and operation of a decision tree has many moving parts, each of which is fairly simple:

(1) select a feature from the full list of predictors;
(2) choose a good cut-point for that feature to split the data into two subgroups;
(3) decide when to stop making new splits in any nodes;
(4) given a terminal node, decide how to classify the next subject that might fall into that node.

Let's consider in detail each of these actions in tree growing.

6.4 Selecting features, making splits

Given data, a tree is generated by first selecting a feature from the full list of features, and the selection occurs at every node under consideration for splitting. Often the feature list is very big: precise genetic evaluations of 500K SNPs for every subject among the 200 in a study, are increasingly common. However, no distributional assumptions or other statistical premises are made in decision trees concerning the features or the subjects.

Selecting a single feature for consideration is done randomly from the full list of predictors. If the list is very long – 500K SNP data for every patient – then the user typically has the option of selecting only some number of the predictors (SNPs) for consideration. This is simply an effort to speed up the computations.

Suppose the full training dataset contains two groups of subjects, Group A and Group B. The goal is to generate a rule that best separates the two groups. Given a feature X, say, possible cut-points for it are evaluated. A *cut-point* for X is a constant, c, and a *split* on this value is of the form $X > c, X \le c$. All subjects having $X > c$ are diverted to one new box (node) and the subjects having $X \le c$ are diverted to another new box (node). Recall Figure 6.1, where the top node was *split* on HDL+LDL $\le$ 240, or $>$ 240.

In what sense is this choice of feature and cut-point any good? If, after making this split using feature X, one of the subsequent (daughter) nodes contains only Group A (at-risk, say) cases, and the other node contains only Group B (not-at-risk) cases, we can probably believe that our split at that node, using that feature, is excellent. The challenge is to define *good* when it's clear that no obviously excellent split is easily available. For this it is convenient to introduce the notion of *purity* in a single node.

6.5 Good split, bad split

Consider an example resulting from a single split, where we start from a single node, Node 1, having 22 Group A cases and 7 Group B cases; see Figure 6.2.

We decide to make a split on some feature, and separate the full group of $22 + 7 = 29$ subjects into two subgroups.

If the new Node 2 has 4 Group A cases, and 5 Group B cases, while the new Node 3 has 18 Group A cases and 2 Group B cases, we can believe that

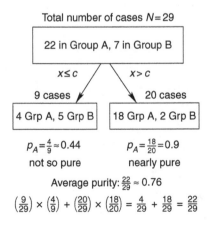

Figure 6.2 A small study in purity.

Node 2 still requires further resolution – more subdivisions – but that Node 3 is close to full resolution. In Node 2 we calculate that the observed Group A rate is 4/9 = 44%, while in Node 3 the rate for Group A is 18/20 = 90%. Using this rate function we say that Node 3 is of higher purity than Node 2. Choosing a cut-point, therefore, and obtaining two nodes such as this results in an *averaged purity* of

$$\frac{9}{20+9} \times \frac{4}{9} + \frac{20}{20+9} \times \frac{18}{20} = \frac{4}{29} + \frac{18}{29} = \frac{22}{29} = 0.759,$$

that is, about 76%. Here the nodes are weighted by the observed (estimated) probability that any data point in the original node gets sent to Node 2, or to Node 3; these weights are, for this example, 9/29 and 20/29.

Let's modify the hypothetical cut-point. We can do this by using the same feature, X, and a different split, $X \leq d$, $X > d$, OR by selecting a different feature, Y, and making a split using that, $Y \leq e$, $Y > e$. Let's suppose we use the same feature and try to find a better split, $X \leq d$, $X > d$. What happens to the within-node and the averaged purity levels? That is, suppose with a different split, we observe that Node 2 has (Group A, Group B) = (11, 2) cases and Node 3 now has (Group A, Group B) = (14, 2) cases; see Figure 6.3.

This yields node purities of

Node 2 = 11/13 = 0.846
Node 3 = 14/16 = 0.875

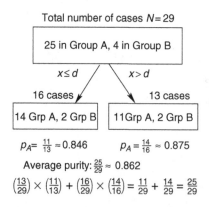

Figure 6.3   Another small study in purity.

and an averaged purity over the two nodes of

average(Node 2, Node 3) = $(11 + 14)/29 = 0.862$.

Our decision to split the data in this single node using a different cut-point (and possibly a different feature as well) has improved on the averaged purity by about 13.6%: an estimated increase in purity from 0.759 to 0.862. We would like to declare such a split as an improvement over our original choice.

Now, the question before us as careful data analysts becomes: is such an improvement statistically and clinically meaningful, or one but not the other, or neither? More precisely, does our choice of purity measure properly quantify our understanding of improvement in this single decision, of how to split the data sitting at this one Node 1?

There are many possible measures of node purity and associated measures of improvement. And the collection of purity measures is still a subject of research. To define some of these purity measures, let's write

p_A = estimated proportion of Group A subjects in a node

p_B = estimated proportion of Group B subjects in a node.

Then three, among many, possible purity measures are:

$\varphi_1(p) = \min(p, 1 - p)$
$\varphi_2(p) = -p \log(p) - (1 - p) \log(1 - p)$
$\varphi_3(p) = p(1 - p)$.

Here we substitute p_A for p in the equations above. It is understood that these purity measures are *estimated* from the sample in a single given node, and that they are node-specific. For example, suppose in a given node we observe four cases belonging to Group A and five belonging to Group B. Then we estimate the Group A fraction as $\hat{p} = 4/9 = 0.444$, and find that these (estimated) purity measures are:

$\varphi_1(0.444) = 0.444$
$\varphi_2(0.444) = 0.298$
$\varphi_3(0.444) = 0.247$.

The lack of equality here tells us that some form of additional practical or theoretical justification is required for selecting a given purity measure.

Moreover, we can also consider how to average, or statistically weight, the estimated node purities for a pair of nodes, using various purity measures.

Here is a justification for the third measure. Let's assign the value 1 to all cases belonging to Group A, and the value 0 to cases in Group B. We think of the result of this assignment at the given node as the outcome of a coin-tossing experiment, where heads = 1 and tails = 0. As a random (binomial) experiment we now compute the sample variance for this experiment and find that

$$\text{sample variance} = \hat{\sigma}^2 = \hat{p}(1 - \hat{p}) = 0.444 \times 0.556 = 0.247.$$

In other words, using purity function φ_3 returns the sample variance for the node. Continuing with this interpretation, minimizing this purity is equivalent to reducing the within-node sample variance. This makes sense: a very pure node should have low sample variance, as the node should contain mostly subjects or instances of the same type. Still further, if we apply the function to a given split of the node into two daughter nodes, and sum over the nodes using the observed weights, we find that the sum is the observed, weighted within-node variance.

This is reminiscent of the within-node variance that we calculate in the analysis of variance, and a good splitting of a single node into two daughter nodes will minimize this variance. So this measure of node purity can be called the *anova* (analysis of variance) measure, but we follow one convention in the classification literature and call it the *Gini index*.

The other measures above, φ_1 and φ_2, have separate justifications, but no purity measure is free from certain anomalies; see the discussion in Section 6.13.

6.6 Finding good features for making splits

Suppose now we have a notion of purity to help us make splits in nodes for a given feature. But what feature do we *finally* select for the split at a given node? One answer is this: use that feature for which the averaged purity of the data at that node improves the most, when evaluated over all features being studied at that given node. Given the differences in purity functions above, a feature that improves one purity function the most at a node, may be different than the feature improving a different purity function, *in that single node*, given the data at that node.

On the other hand, it is our experience that most splitting rules, and associated purity functions, eventually lead to very similar classifying engines. The conclusion of all the chosen possible splits – the fully grown tree – is what really matters, and this is measured by the usual summary accuracy values: error, sensitivity, specificity.

There is a basic tree idea at work here: how a tree *looks*, complex, simple or something in between, is not a reliable indication of its predictive ability. To make this point clearer let's look at an apparently easy decision problem.

6.7 Misreading trees

Sample data for a relatively simple decision problem is given in Figure 6.4(a), (b), and (c).

By construction, the true decision boundary is slightly curved, but is not that complicated. Making a single cut on the X-axis does not seem to help much, nor does a single cut on the Y-axis. Still it would be a mistake to suppose that any *initial* single cut on either feature is representative of the predictive capacity of a fully grown tree on this data. The tops of trees are basically not relevant to good decision-making; it's the bottoms that matter.

Let's look at this problem more closely. In Figure 6.5(a), (b) a series of cuts have been made, using both X and Y. Another series of cuts have been made in Figure 6.6(a), (b), and (c).

The trees corresponding to these splits in Figures 6.5 and 6.6, are closely related yet also very different. Let's observe the following about these trees:

(1) The decision boundaries for the two trees are identical.
(2) Equally good trees can look very different.
(3) The data included in the individual nodes of the two trees are not the same.
(4) The first split at the top of the trees are different.

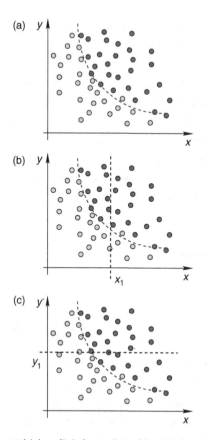

Figure 6.4   Which split is better? And in which order?

(5) The actual cut-points for the splits are the same but they appear in a different order in the two trees. The split at x_1 appears at the top of the tree in Figure 6.6(a), and appears at the third level in the tree in Figure 6.6(b).

(6) Observe that the decision regions for these two trees, when pooled across similar regions, are identical. Thus the decision region *jointly* covered by Boxes 1, 3, 5, and 6 in Figure 6.5(c) is identical to the decision region *jointly* covered by Boxes 1, 3, 5, and 6 in Figure 6.6(c). Neighboring boxes can generate the same decision.

We strongly urge caution in interpreting tree structure. These are basically simple, often compelling gadgets, with not-so-simple logic.

Given that many splits may be required for data, let's next consider how to *stop* making splits.

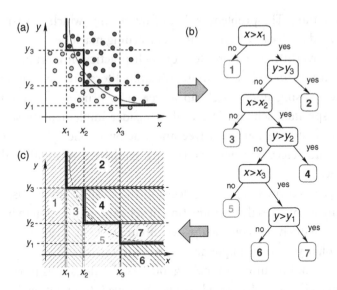

Figure 6.5   One way to slice up the data. (See plate section for color version.)

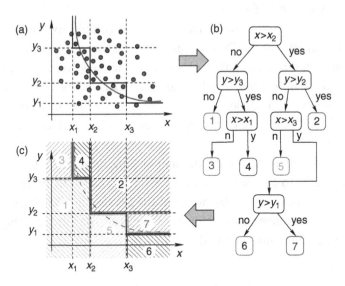

Figure 6.6   Another way to slice up the data; or is it? (See plate section for color version.)

6.8 Stopping and pruning rules

Rules for stopping can be straightforward. One simple result, after a sequence of earlier splits, is a node with just one or a few cases remaining. It is generally inefficient to continue trying to split a node with just, say, five cases remaining. The problem is that of overfitting, which is a larger issue and a hazard for basically any statistical learning machine.

Indeed, overfitting is a problem of such practical importance that, for decision trees, there is a separate research literature on *pruning* trees, that is, collapsing nodes back up a tree. The pruning process is not a uniquely specified scheme. We could consider implementing some node collapsing over one part of a tree and not over other parts of the tree. Or we could select one node collapsing method over another throughout a tree.

One early scheme for pruning decision trees, with some statistical logic supporting it, involves the introduction of yet another function to be defined on a tree, namely its *complexity*; see Breiman *et al.* (1993). Under this pruning plan we would implement a decision tree that had only sufficient complexity (and no more) to make good classifications. It is possible that a more involved, more elaborated tree might have interpretational problems, and also important is the argument that an unnecessarily complex tree is more likely to overfit the data.

Further aspects of pruning trees and tree complexity lead into more theoretical questions; see DGL (chapter 20). Theory suggests that any classification method, or any family of learning machines, has a model richness, a so-called *VC dimension*, by which its complexity can be evaluated; see the earlier discussion in Section 2.7. We note that for now it is not clear how Breiman's notion of tree complexity connects with or differs from the VC dimension.

Theory also suggests that the number of subjects appearing in any terminal node needs to be monitored as the sample grows. The practical view of this is: for a given sample size, we want the amount of available data in the terminal nodes to give a good estimate of the *local* group membership for any future cases falling into that node.

6.9 Using functions of the features

So far we have only considered splitting on single features, and for these we have only looked at splits using constants and inequalities, things of the form $X \leq c$, or $X > c$.

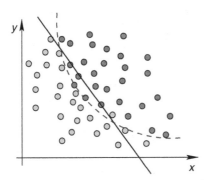

Figure 6.7   Why not use a single, probably better split, something other than a vertical or horizontal line?

See the data given in Figure 6.4 again. As we saw, for such data a single split using X or Y does not generate a good decision rule. And a single, very simple function of the features could do much better than any single splits of the form $X \leq c$ $X > c$ or $Y \leq d$, $Y > d$. This is clear from Figure 6.7.

It is also clear that a linear function of the data might often do better *locally* when compared to many splits of these simple types. But this also does not undermine the utility of the complex trees that are grown and never use any linear (sloping-line) function.

That a good linear summary score can *initially* do better than the raw scores on which it is based, but do less well than the raw scores themselves, is a phenomenon we've seen before. Thus, the summary comorbidity measures – Charlson and SLE morbidity in the lupus data analysis of Chapter 4 – outperformed the raw scores when both the summaries and the raw scores were in the model. However, the two summaries did less well when compared to feature lists that included *only* the raw scores. This is also related to the problem we discussed in Chapter 5 on calibration for logistic regression. Thus, using a summary measure inside another model is effectively using one machine inside another, and we need to be alert to the possibility that error values can in this case go up *or* down.

6.10 Unstable trees?

As we have seen above, growing a single decision tree can lead to overfitting, and then lead to poor results when applied to new data: the tree is said to not

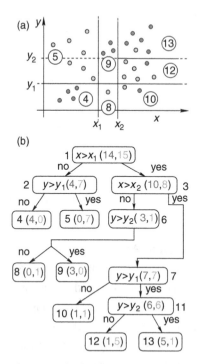

Figure 6.8   Splitting to near purity.

generalize very well. Let's look at this problem more carefully. Our remarks here apply to statistical learning machines generally, and are not meant to be specifically critical of single decision trees.

Consider fitting a tree scheme to the data in Figure 6.8(a), (b). After several, entirely plausible splits we find that the data in the individual smaller rectangles each contain essentially only one group of cases, either those of Group *A* or those of Group *B*.

On the other hand, the cases in the smallest rectangles are typically few in number. Hence, where we have observed two cases of Group *A* in a cell, we would declare any new case, falling into this cell and having unknown group membership, to be classified as Group *A*. This means that over this tree, we are in fact looking at terminal nodes – decision cells – that are only thinly represented. An alternative to the many small cells is a tree with many fewer nodes, as in Figure 6.9(a) with its tree in Figure 6.9(b).

Such local instability is one version of the overfitting problem. Given a small sample size in a terminal node, we expect a high sample variance for

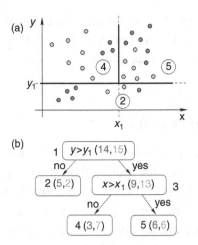

Figure 6.9   Fewer splits, less purity, but also less overfitting and better prediction.

any statistical estimation in that node, which then translates into an unstable classifier for any subject appearing in the node.

There is, however, another kind of instability that also requires attention. Namely, results from tree theory report that the local boxes generated in the tree building *must* be unstable in the sense that they must be allowed to adapt to the data as it increases. This makes practical sense since the local boxes should predict group membership increasingly well as data accumulates, and this is only done by shifting the walls of the local boxes – or splitting up over-stuffed boxes into smaller ones. Note here, too, that a single tree (or forest for that matter) is *not* guaranteed by theory to be optimal unless it gets the opportunity to shift the walls as data is gathered. Re-estimating the box walls as data is gathered is in fact a standard data analysis process: we don't expect a simple linear regression to approximate the true regression line arbitrarily well if it isn't allowed to shift about as the sample increases.

Studying the data and the trees in this example, it might seem that all three are overfitting the data, by following the apparent decision boundary much too closely. This may or may not be true, and we can't know for sure until relatively far down the road towards validation of the decision rule; see Chapter 11.

That is, overfitting might be thought to occur primarily when the cell sample sizes of the terminal nodes in a tree are too small. Having small cells can certainly suggest overfitting, but in fact, what are the cell sizes in the two trees in

Figure 6.5(a) and (b)? These are not obviously small – the terminal nodes all seem well populated. Thus, the practical conclusion here is that apparent overfitting cannot be so easily judged by inspection of local boundary tracking.

6.11 Variable importance – growing on trees?

Just above, we criticized the misreading of trees. This occurs when we might be inclined to think of the first few variable choices, those at the top of a tree, as a reflection of the overall, empirical usefulness of those features. We presented examples that reveal this approach as mistaken. Later, in Chapter 9, in the sections on interpreting coefficients in small models, we will urge caution in how *those* coefficients might be seen as measures of variable importance. However, we have not pointed to any set of methods that could be offered as reliable alternatives. Let's take up this question again now, in the context of growing decision trees, and discuss some possible, positive answers.

The central problem is this – in language suggestive of more formal mathematics – the contribution any single feature makes to a model is not a well-posed question. And it probably can't be well posed in the specific context of biomedical research. What procedures or drugs we choose to apply to a given medical condition are, sensibly, nearly always context-dependent. The statistical restatement of this biomedical reality is that the usefulness of any single feature is a highly nontrivial function of all the other features already appearing in the model, or indeed, of those features we should have measured but didn't. Indeed, it is possible that the basic variable importance problem, for a given large set of features, may not be optimally resolved in any practical time frame: this is a monster.

And the variable importance problem is closely related to the question of *interactions* between features – but this is also not a well-posed problem mathematically. Consider the data and trees in Figure 6.10.

The data has been split in two ways, using y first, and then x, and the other way round, x first and then y. The decision rule for the next subject is the same; the error rates are apparently the same. The features here need to cooperate in some way, and this cooperation is not well assessed using feature selection order.

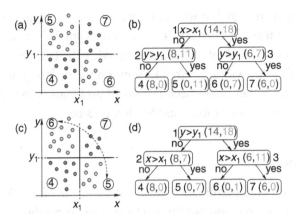

Figure 6.10   Two ways to split the data. Order and ranking relationships in interacting features can be hard to sort out.

It is interesting to note here that we could achieve virtually the same decision boundary and apparent error rate by introducing a single new function: the product of x and y. Just as we saw in Chapter 5 when we introduced a multiplicative interaction term for the logistic regression model, and a decision rule was generated using two (so-called) branches of a hyperbola. In that cholesterol example one of the branches (in the lower right of Figures 5.2, 5.3, and 5.4) was deep into the at-risk zone yet the decision rule would automatically declare every subject landing there as not at risk. Using both branches of the hyperbola was a mistake for that data. On the other hand, it is seen with not too much effort that using both branches of a fitted hyperbola would do really well for the data in Figure 6.10. Otherwise expressed, the familiar multiplicative interaction term in a model may be an advance or a hazard.

Still it makes sense to attempt ranking the importance of features, given that we are eyes wide open about the hazards.

Assume that we have arrived at a node in a single decision tree, and that we want to further divide it. Assume that we also want to estimate the relative usefulness of any of the features, *at this node.* We can use the Gini index of node purity for this. Each feature will induce a reduction in Gini purity in its individual attempt to split the given node. We can, therefore, list the Gini purity reductions for each, and order them least to greatest. The node-splitting method that uses the Gini index will split using the feature having the largest purity reduction, but we can record all the other Gini reductions as well. Then, it is feasible to consider the average Gini reduction over the entire tree that is generated by each feature. Ranking the tree averages, over all the nodes, then provides a variable importance ordering for all the features. But recently there have been reports of problems with this simple and intuitive approach: see Note 3, and Section 6.13 below.

6.12 Permuting for importance

We introduce a variable permutation idea that can be used for the importance of any feature, a method not limited to tree-based machines. It seems to be more reliable and not subject to some of the problems reported for the Gini index.

Consider drawing a bootstrap sample from the data (for which see Chapter 10), and keeping track of the subjects *not* included in the draw. Breiman *et al.* (1993), introduced the OOB notation for these not-included subjects. We can now train any given method on the bootstrap draw which serves as training data, and then generate an estimate of its accuracy by testing it on the cases not included in the bootstrap draw, the OOB sample.

Suppose, however, that instead of using the OOB cases exactly as given, we select one of the features in the model, more specifically, let's suppose we are studying a single feature in the cholesterol data, LDL. We replace its appearance in all the OOB cases with a "noisy" version of itself. That is, we list all the values of LDL that appear in every OOB subject, and that there are six subjects that are OOB. Suppose further that the full list of all LDL cholesterol levels for all six OOB subjects is {101, 95, 165, 186, 120, 98}. Then a permuted *reordering* of these values could be {98, 186, 165, 95, 101, 120}. In this reordering the values of the other feature, HDL, of each subject that are OOB remain the same, including the known outcome for each subject. The values of LDL for each OOB subject have been rendered noisy; the value for HDL is unchanged.

We proceed to evaluate the estimated error in classifying each OOB subject, where we have replaced, for each subject, its permuted LDL value. Thus, the first subject, instead of having LDL = 101, now has an assigned LDL = 98; the second subject, instead of having LDL = 95, now has LDL = 186, etc.

The next step in evaluating the importance of LDL using this permutation method is calculation of the difference in estimated error values, using the real data and then using the permuted LDL data.

We can do this permutation and error estimation at every node in the tree, as it is grown, and then take averages over all the nodes in the tree. Finally, we order the features according to their average changes in error values. If the permuted version of a given feature produces little change in the average error estimate then we argue that this feature is, really, not much different from noise. If the permuted version of the feature produces a large difference in the average error estimate then presumably this feature has relatively high information content. In this way a permutation of the values of a single feature will generate a ranking in importance for each feature.

The permutation method is not limited to gauging feature importance as part of a decision tree. It is, in our opinion, an excellent method for biomedical data for estimating the importance of any decision rule; see Chapter 11. For a slightly different version of the permutation method for evaluating the importance of features in a logistic regression model, see Potter (2005, 2008).

Finally, a permutation method as above will generate a list of feature importances. Several questions then arise:

(1) How good is this list? Do the top members of the list really do better than those lower down?
(2) If we start with another but similar dataset, would we get the same list? How stable is this list?
(3) Given another ranking of features, how do we combine them into a single, better list?

These are all questions currently under intensive research. The problem of ranking generally is discussed in Section 9.7.

6.13 The continuing mystery of trees

Methods for calculating variable importances and understanding trees keep bubbling along in the research literature. Some of the earlier methods are now clearly seen to behave in odd ways: see Strobl *et al.* (2008), Nicodemus *et al.* (2009, 2010). In these studies it was shown how Random Forests, when using the Gini index for variable importances, consistently selects features *at the first splits* in all trees that have a positive connection with other features. This is *feature–feature* correlation here, to be distinguished from the correlation of a feature with the outcome to be predicted.

Indeed, in Nicodemus and Malley (2009), it was shown that if the data had *no* signal at all then features that are uncorrelated with other features were much more likely to be selected at the first split in all trees. Moreover, in Nicodemus *et al.* (2010), it was found that if the data had a strong signal (using simulated data from a linear model) then features that were correlated with others were more likely to be selected at the first split, under the Gini option.

An important note about these recent findings is: what a tree does at the very top is almost certainly not a good way to assess how it does by the time it gets to the bottom. And it is only at the bottom, where the terminal nodes appear, that the tree is making decisions on new cases. Looking at just the tops of a tree is also certainly not a good way to assess how it assigns variable importances. That is, overall tree or forest performance should be evaluated in terms of estimated errors, either prediction errors or approximate mean square errors (in the regression case). And the *order* in which a tree (or forest) goes about splitting up the sample space into tiny boxes is unrelated to the size or placement of the boxes themselves.

For the two studies above, error values were either not good (in the case of no signal, as we should expect) or were quite good (in the case of a strong signal). Hence these trees generally behaved as expected as prediction engines and as systems for grading variable importances, regardless of the correlations between the predictors themselves.

On the other hand, examples exist where we can't remove correlation structure in the data. A single SNP embedded in a block of other SNPs with high linkage disequilibrium (LD) may be the causative SNP, or in the causative gene. Here high LD should not deter selection. In fact, for SNPs close to the causative SNP or gene it may not be biologically meaningful to think of the SNP as separable from the causative SNP or gene: evolution has not had time or reason to separate this LD block. For such data, correlations between features is not something that requires removal or adjustment. Indeed, it may not make biological sense to discount the existing correlation structure. This leads to the deeper problem of motif and genetic network detection; see Chapter 13.

7

Random Forests – trees everywhere

The clearest path into the Universe is through a forest wilderness.

John Muir

The world's a forest, in which all lose their way;
though by a different path each goes astray.

George Villiers

Having discussed single decision trees we move on to large collections of trees and Random Forests, RF. As a single scheme this began as a collection of methods smartly pulled together by Leo Breiman and Adele Cutler. They built on previous work, for example in doing bootstrap draws from the data upon which to train single trees, and also helped promote the novel idea of randomly sampling from the list of features; see Note 1.

RF continues to demonstrate excellent performance on a wide range of data. Currently it is our preferred learning machine, for its speed, convenience, and generally good performance.

7.1 Random Forests in less than five minutes

Here is an outline of the Random Forests procedure.

(1) Sample the data, using bootstrap draws; keep track of the data selected, and call the data *not* selected the (OOB) out-of-bag data; recall that bootstrap sampling means sampling *with* replacement.

(2) Sample the list of features; here we don't sample with replacement (as in boot draws), choosing in each draw only a small number of the features from the complete list (this small number is, basically, the main user-specified parameter for the whole RF scheme).

(3) Grow a single decision tree using the data and features selected; don't bother with pruning or finding the optimal size or complexity of the tree.

(4) For this single tree above, use the OOB data to estimate the error value of the tree.

(5) Do steps (1) through (4) again (and again); the default number of repetitions is often 500, but more can be grown if necessary; the collection of trees is called a *random forest*.

(6) To classify a new case drop it down all the trees in the forest, and take the simple majority vote across all trees to make a decision for that case.

There continue to be additions and important refinements to the scheme above, but RF is basically just that simple; see also Strobl *et al.* (2008, 2009). It is not clear from this description why such a simple method should prove to be proficient in so many practical applications to biomedical (and other) data. We take up this question shortly, but let's go over the steps in more detail.

7.2 Random treks through the data

In our previous discussion of bootstrap sampling we remarked upon two important features of this scheme.

First, each boot draw can be seen as representative, in a statistical sense, of the original population, so that multiple boot draws can ultimately (in sufficiently large samples, etc.) closely approximate the original population from which they are all drawn.

Second, while the data chosen in a boot draw can be used for estimation, the data *not* chosen in a boot draw can also be used for an important task, that of evaluating the goodness of the estimate just made. That is, the OOB data serves as a surrogate for new data which is also considered as representative of the original population.

Neither of these approaches to data analysis is new in the statistical literature. However, there is a further innovation in RF that is parallel to bootstrapping from the data, and that significantly enhances the data resampling approach. We now discuss this.

7.3 Random treks through the features

We have commented on the problem of *context* for the predictive power of any single predictor, so that the power of a feature was shown to be highly contingent on the other features in the model. We have also noted that given a long list of possible features it can be especially difficult to select any verifiably good subset of features. Indeed, as noted earlier, the problem of making an optimal selection from among a very big list of features is probably not solvable in any reasonable computing time.

The RF scheme deals with this problem as it does with the data itself, by repeated sampling. Specifically, from the complete list of features we select a small subset, by sampling without replacement; see Note 2.

Thus, given the features {*a, b, c, d,* ..., *x, y, z*}, a single selection could, for example, yield the subset {*a, b, c, x, y*}. In these selections it is understood that we usually take a small fraction of the total number of features: the default is the square root of the total size of the feature list, so for a list of 26 features (the alphabet list just given) we make a random selection of five features: $\sqrt{26} \approx 5$. This choice is not certain to be optimal for every data set, and RF tries to optimize it somewhat by moving up or down slightly from the default of the square root of the sample size. The size of this draw is a user input. In our experience this doesn't yield a significant increase in predictive capacity of any forest, but should still be considered an option to explore.

But, why should we be interested in looking at only a tiny, short list of features in building a decision tree, or indeed in a tiny list that is constantly changing? An answer is related to our discussion of context for each feature. By choosing randomly from the full feature list, and for each selection building many trees, we are, in effect, looking at an average over all the contexts in which a given feature can occur. This is a smoothing, therefore, across the feature context landscape. Moreover, it often results in multiple feature lists that generate models that are relatively uncorrelated with each other, and this we show in Chapter 11 is known to produce good performance overall.

Finally, we observe that the random subspace method has recently been applied to improve performance of boosting schemes; see Garcia-Pedrajas and Ortiz-Boyer (2008).

7.4 Walking through the forest

Having discussed the basic mechanisms of RF, random sampling from the data and from the list of features, we now describe the scheme as a whole, and focus on the two-group classification problem.

(1) Begin by doing a boot draw from the data; if the groups are approximately equal in size then the draw will result in two groups also approximately equal in size (for unequal groups see below); keep track of the cases not selected, and call these the OOB cases.

(2) Generate a single tree using the selected (in-bag) cases, using this method:

    (2a) at each node randomly select m features from the complete list of features – a standard default is $m \approx \sqrt{M}$, where M is the total number of features;

    (2b) using the m selected features find that feature and its optimal cut-point, that minimizes the Gini error, or the average decrease in error – make a split using that (locally) optimal feature;

    (2c) proceed to the next nodes and repeat steps (2a) and (2b) above – grow the tree until some halting rule is satisfied, typically this is when the node contains just a few (say, 5) cases or less.

(3) With a single tree grown to maximum size, drop all the OOB cases down the tree and track the terminal node for each such case; classify the case by majority vote in the terminal node.

(4) Repeat steps (1), (2), (3) and generate more trees; typically 500.

(5) Use the majority vote across all the trees to classify each case (weighted voting methods are also possible); generate error rates (along with sensitivity and specificity estimates).

Steps (1) through (5) will produce a set of trees, a *forest*, and generally good estimates of the error rate for the forest. It is the forest *as a whole* that constitutes the Random Forests algorithm: the collection of all trees is the "model."

7.5 Weighted and unweighted voting

We have described the RF procedure using a method for classifying each case by a simple majority vote across the trees in the forest. This is a sound and generally satisfactory method for many datasets. However, there is one situation that is recurrent in biomedical data analysis, that for which the numbers of cases in the two groups under study are unequal, say for data having 25 patients and 250 controls. As we have mentioned before, most perfectly good learning machines, when presented with such group imbalance, will decide to classify most cases as controls rather than patients, and thereby lower the average error rate. However, the average lowering comes at a cost, in that the error values for the smaller group go up, often substantially. That is, the sensitivity for the method blows up. We have discussed this before; we believe it bears repetition.

Blowing up like this is not good, unless there is some biomedical or clinical reason for allowing such increases. There may be, for example, misclassification costs or disease prevalence rates that justify an imbalance between sensitivity and specificity. We discuss this balancing problem more completely in Chapter 11.

Therefore, in the absence of some well-stated *scientific* reason for seeking unequal sensitivity and specificity rates we choose to try and balance the rates; see Chapter 11. We outline three methods for doing this.

Method 1: Define an alternative voting scheme, in which we don't use a simple majority vote across the trees, but instead make the group assignment with a cut-point of something other than 50% (the majority vote rule). Breiman and Cutler (see the RF website) have implemented in their version of RF a method that lets the user assign a vote weight, so that a case, for example, might be put in the patient group if 75% or more of the trees in the forest put the case in that group. In the example above, where the group sizes had a ratio of 10 to 1, they would recommend starting the balancing process using a weight of 10.

However, the selection of voting weight based on *just* the observed group ratio is not statistically guaranteed to balance the error rates, and we recommend using this weight as a tuning parameter. It is possible to be more systematic than just using an input weight equal to the group ratio, by making multiple runs with varying weight settings and calculating the observed rates. In our experience, when the datasets are relatively small, such as, indeed, the 25 patients and 250 controls datasets, we have found that the tuning process is not very stable and hard to interpret. Thus, the estimated optimal weight might be 15.7 and not 15.78, even for the 25/250 dataset. This possibly time-consuming tuning process therefore strikes us as neither practical nor theoretically well-understood.

Method 2: Simply send fully balanced datasets to RF for processing. This total prebalancing is easy to do and guarantees that the estimated error values will be balanced. This is our preferred method. We can create balanced datasets by first bootstrapping from the two groups, using a sample size equal to the size of the smaller of the two groups. This is the data balancing method called *down-sampling*, or *under-sampling* (from the larger group). The prebalancing is done repeatedly, and RF is given in each instance the prebalanced data.

Method 3: We need to mention one more method for equalizing the error rates, a scheme that appears in the R code version of RF, as the *sampsize* option. With this option selected and the size of the smaller group chosen as the sampsize, the method works as follows:

(a) a bootstrap sample is drawn from each group, of $n = sampsize$;
(b) the RF program then constructs a forest in the usual way, but then
(c) it tests each case that is OOB on the cases not selected in the original draw.

This method seems sound enough but there is a problem. That is, after the first boot draw, the remaining cases form two groups with a size ratio that is different from the original group ratio. This means, therefore, that the case testings (predictions) are done on groups that are not representative in relative sizes to the original groups.

As an illustration, suppose the two groups are of size 25 and 300. A boot draw of size 25 will select about two-thirds of the patients, that is about 16 cases, and about two-thirds of the controls, that is about about 200 cases. Thus we now have a group ratio of 12.5, not $300/25 = 12$. When the groups are both smaller, the discrepancy is more pronounced. When presented with grossly unequal sample sizes, most learning machines can be expected to make this standard mistake, by limiting the overall error rate by classifying most cases as members of the larger group at the expense of the smaller one.

7.6 Finding subsets in the data using proximities

We now discuss how random forests as constructed by Breiman and Cutler include yet another innovation – this scheme really does have many moving parts. Namely, it smoothly includes *multidimensional scaling* (MDS) plots based on distances between subjects as estimated by RF.

MDS is a huge subject with a long history, technical and practical; see Borg and Groenen (2005), Cox and Cox (2001). We already discussed the basics of MDS in Section 2.4. Here is a quick review.

First, between every pair of the objects of study (in our case, subjects) we introduce some notion of distance between the objects. As every pair of objects then has a calculated distance, the list of pairwise counts can grow quickly as more objects are introduced. To put the pairwise counts into the form of a *distance function*, a transformation is required; see Note 3.

Second, the collection of pairwise distances is further transformed so as to highlight or concentrate the essential variation in the list of distances. This proceeds exactly as in principal component analysis.

The question now is: How can we get subject–subject, pairwise distances using trees? Here is one method: for a given pair of subjects count the number of times they appear together in any terminal node in any tree. It is argued that if they appear together this way quite often then they are closer than other subject–subject pairings.

Given the transformed paired distances, the principal component transformation returns a list of the top most-varying dimensions in the component space. It is the case that the simple Euclidean distances between subjects in these top-most dimensions is approximately the same as their original transformed distance.

Subjects appearing close together may or may not be in the same classes, Group *A* or Group *B*, but we would expect to see the Group *A* subjects closer to each other than the Group *B* subjects. Such clustering tells us approximately how well the groups are being separated by the RF procedure (or in fact, by any other machine), but there are two key ideas also at work here:

(1) Some subjects in Group *A* can be closer to parts of Group *B* than they are to other Group *A* subjects. This suggests some less-than-obvious commonality in these subsets. Since each subject is uniquely identified in these MDS plots, we can go back and study the clinical or biological record to see why this might occur.

(2) The clustering evidenced in these MDS plots is based on using all the predictors as chosen by RF in its tree-building activities. If we witness

distinct subsets of subjects in the MDS plots we can ask: is it possible that the subsets might be better separated by using different lists, that is sublists of predictors, where the sublists were not necessarily selected as most important by the original forest in its attempt to model the data. Simply put, it is plausible that one subset of subjects might be better separated from other subsets of subjects, by using different sets of predictors. Having identified possible subsets of subjects it might be useful to see if RF can be more accurate as a prediction engine when it is given just that subset upon which to work. This process is an example of cycling from a supervised learning machine, RF, to an unsupervised machine, MDS, and then back to a supervised one, RF, again, now acting on a different subset. Such cycling is not limited to RF and clustering through MDS plots: it is to be encouraged when using machines quite generally.

7.7 Applying Random Forests to the Stroke data

We apply Random Forests to the Stroke-A dataset. Recall the details from Chapter 4. There are 49 features, and among patients with no missing data, there were 933 patients who experienced complete restitution and 479 patients who did not. Thus, the data is unbalanced, so we apply RF using a prebalanced dataset, using the under-sampling method, as described above. Let's start by recalling the basics of this dataset.

Definitions

Groups are defined by the Barthel Index total score after 90 days (v394):

Group 1 = Complete restitution: v394 ≥ 95
Group 0 = Partial restitution: v394 < 95.
Subjects who died were excluded from the analysis.

The analysis of the training dataset goes as follows.

Training results

The larger group (complete restitution) was randomly sampled without replacement to a size equal to the smaller group (partial restitution). The

Table 7.1 Mean errors on training data averaged over all forests, ± 2 Std errors

OOB	23.7 (23.7, 23.8)
Group 0	23.1 (23.0, 23.2)
Group 1	24.4 (24.3, 24.4)

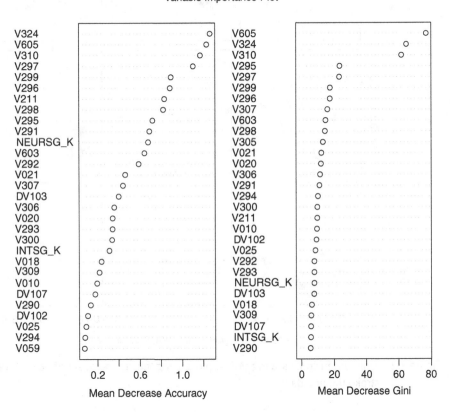

Figure 7.1   Variable importance plots for all 38 features, using training data.

total N analyzed was 1114, with 557 in each group. The analysis file had 38 candidate predictor variables. The analysis included 100 forests, each with 1000 trees. (Software versions were R version 2.9.2 (2009–08–24), randomForest 4.5–33.)

The mean error rates are given in Table 7.1.

Next, we use the first forest (in the set of 100) to generate a variable importance plot, shown in Figure 7.1, and a multidimensional scaling plot

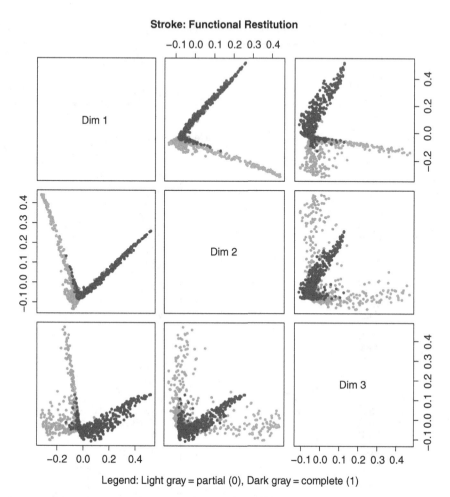

Figure 7.2 Multidimensional scaling (MDS) plots using the complete set of 38 features for the stroke training data.

(discussed in Section 2.4), shown in Figure 7.2. Next we calculated standardized variable importances, averaged over the 100 forests, as shown in Table 7.2.

Using the mean decrease in accuracy method for determining feature importance, we select the top 10 features and do RF again. Notice that we recover more subjects with complete data using the smaller feature list, so that there are 557 patients who had complete restitution and 1019 patients who did not. The error rates are given in Table 7.3.

Table 7.2 Variable importance rankings for all 38 features standardized to 0–100 scale and averaged over all forests

Variable	Description	Mean decrease in accuracy (± 2 Std errors)
v324	Functional impairment (Rankin) at 48–72 hrs	98.9 (98.5, 99.2)
v310	Baseline NIHSS[1] total score	98.0 (97.5, 98.6)
v605	Age at event in years	66.6 (66.2, 66.9)
v297	Baseline NIHSS best motor right arm	46.7 (46.4, 47.0)
v299	Baseline NIHSS motor right leg	31.0 (30.7, 31.3)
v296	Baseline NIHSS best motor left arm	27.7 (27.4, 28.0)
v298	Baseline NIHSS motor left leg	21.2 (20.9, 21.4)
v295	Baseline NIHSS facial palsy	21.1 (20.8, 21.3)
v291	Baseline NIHSS questions	18.3 (18.0, 18.5)
v603	Gender	15.5 (15.3, 15.7)
v211	Fever > 38°C within 72 hrs	13.4 (13.3, 13.5)
v292	Baseline NIHSS commands	10.9 (10.7, 11.0)
v307	Baseline NIHSS dysarthria	9.9 (9.7, 10.1)
v021	Diabetes mellitus	9.4 (9.2, 9.5)
neursg_k	Neurological complications within 72 hrs	7.1 (7.0, 7.2)
v306	Baseline NIHSS best language	7.1 (6.9, 7.2)
v020	Arterial hypertension	5.9 (5.7, 6.0)
dv103	Local to lenticulostriate arteries	5.4 (5.2, 5.5)
v300	Baseline NIHSS limb ataxia	4.6 (4.5, 4.7)
v293	Baseline NIHSS best gaze	3.7 (3.6, 3.8)
v010	Prior stroke: history of prior stroke	3.3 (3.2, 3.4)
v309	Baseline NIHSS extinction/inattention	2.9 (2.8, 3.0)
intsg_k	Other medical complications	2.7 (2.7, 2.8)
v018	Prior peripheral arterial disease	2.4 (2.3, 2.5)
dv107	Local to brain stem arteries	2.1 (2.1, 2.2)
dv102	Local to middle cerebral artery	1.8 (1.6, 1.9)
v290	Baseline NIHSS level of consciousness	1.7 (1.6, 1.8)
v305	Baseline NIHSS sensory	1.7 (1.6, 1.9)
v025	Smoking	1.3 (1.2, 1.4)
v059	Lowering of elevated blood glucose	1.3 (1.2, 1.4)
v294	Baseline NIHSS visual	1.2 (1.1, 1.3)
dv104	Local to thalamic arteries	0.8 (0.7, 0.9)

Table 7.2 (cont.)

Variable	Description	Mean decrease in accuracy (± 2 Std errors)
dv108	Local to middle/posterior cerebral arteries	0.8 (0.8, 0.9)
dv109	Local to anterior/middle cerebral arteries	0.7 (0.7, 0.8)
dv101	Local to anterior cerebral artery	0.6 (0.5, 0.6)
dv110	Local to long perforating arteries	0.6 (0.6, 0.7)
dv105	Local to posterior cerebral artery	0.3 (0.3, 0.4)
dv106	Local to cerebellar arteries	0.1 (0.0, 0.1)

[1] National Institutes of Health Stroke Scale.

Table 7.3. Mean error, top 10 features on training data averaged over all forests, ± 2 Std errors

OOB	26.4 (26.3, 26.4)
Group 0	26.7 (26.6, 26.8)
Group 1	26.0 (26.0, 26.1)

The variable importances using just the top 10 features are presented in Figure 7.3 and in Table 7.4.

Note that the ordering of the features in the top 10 list is not precisely the same as in the listing for all 38 features: v310 and v 324 are switched, while the arm and leg features get sorted differently as well. This is an example of two processes:

(1) variable importance is a function of the other variables under consideration, in this case the full list of 38 and the reduced list of just 10;
(2) importance rankings are inherently unstable, for more on this foundational problem see Section 9.7.

Evidently using just the top 10 features results in error drift, from about 23.7% (using all 38 features) to 26.4%. Next, we display the MDS plots for the top 10 features, Figure 7.4.

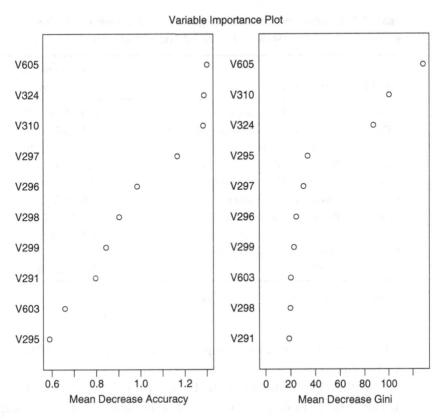

Figure 7.3   Variable importance plots using the top 10 features on the training data.

Careful inspection of the MDS plots, those for all 38 features and those for the top 10 features, and the table of error rates, tells the same story: there is more overlap in the two groups using a smaller feature list. That is, the two groups, complete or partial restitution, are harder to separate using only the top 10 features. It is good practice to check that the two methods of presenting the RF results – error table and MDS plot – report similar outcomes.

Finally we apply RF to the Stroke-B data, which we use as a validation step. For this we use the first forest generated in the set of 100, and all 38 features. The error rates are given in Table 7.5. The first forest resulting from the training file analysis, using all 38 features, was applied to the Stroke-B dataset. The *predict* function in randomForest was invoked, and prior to testing the prediction, the group sizes in the validation file were

Table 7.4. Variable importance rankings for top 10 features on training data standardized to 0–100 scale and averaged over all 100 forests

Variable	Description	Mean decrease in accuracy (± 2 Std errors)
V310	Baseline NIHSS[2] total score	100.0 (100.0, 100.0)
V324	Functional impairment (Rankin) at 48–72 hrs	76.3 (75.7, 76.9)
V605	Age at event in years	65.6 (65.1, 66.0)
V297	Baseline NIHSS best motor right arm	41.8 (41.4, 42.1)
V296	Baseline NIHSS best motor left arm	19.0 (18.7, 19.3)
V299	Baseline NIHSS motor right leg	13.6 (13.3, 13.9)
V298	Baseline NIHSS motor left leg	9.3 (9.0, 9.5)
V291	Baseline NIHSS questions	6.0 (5.7, 6.3)
V295	Baseline NIHSS facial palsy	1.6 (1.3, 1.8)
V603	Gender	0.3 (0.2, 0.4)

[2] National Institutes of Health Stroke Scale.

equalized to 680 in each group with random sampling (Precision = 1– Error rate).

Next, the top 10 features were applied to the validation (Stroke-B) dataset, as displayed in Table 7.6. The first forest resulting from the training file analysis, using 10 features, was applied to the Stroke-B dataset. The *predict* function in randomForest was invoked, and prior to testing the prediction, the group sizes in the validation file were equalized to 680 in each group with random sampling (Precision = 1– Error rate).

We compare the validation results using all 38 features and just the top 10. We find a slight error drift between the training data for both feature sets, and also a drift from the training data to the validation data. In Chapter 11 we show how to rigorously compare the two error rates, derived from applying two machines to the same validation, independent dataset.

The results obtained above can also be compared with those found in König *et al.* (2007). Note that we only used 38 of the full list of 43 features studied there, as we needed to have data that was complete in all features, in both datasets, in order to apply the machines to Stroke A and Stroke B.

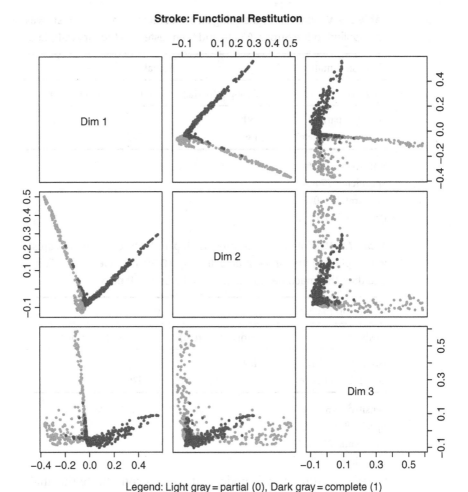

Figure 7.4   MDS plots using the top 10 features.

7.8 Random Forests in the universe of machines

The Random Forests machine, and the collection of submethods it contains, is one machine among many. In our experience it does quite well, but recall the warning we gave in Chapter 1: there are no super-classifiers. For any given machine there exists a dataset and another machine that must provably do better than our original machine.

On the theory side, RF is still not fully understood. Its many moving parts – bootstrap draws from the data, draws from the feature list, cut-points

Table 7.5 Validation results using all 38 features. Random Forests was first applied to the Stroke-A data and then tested on the Stroke-B data

Confusion matrix	Actual	
Predicted	Group 0 (partial)	Group 1 (complete)
Group 0 (partial)	491	151
Group 1 (complete)	189	529

Sensitivity: 72.2%
Specificity: 77.8%
Error rate: 25.0%
Precision: 75.0%

Table 7.6 Validation results using the top 10 features. Random Forests was applied to the Stroke-A data, the top 10 features were identified, and then this machine was applied to the Stroke-B data

Confusion matrix	Actual	
Predicted	Group 0 (partial)	Group 1 (complete)
Group 0 (partial)	464	155
Group 1 (complete)	216	525

Sensitivity: 68.2%
Specificity: 77.2%
Error rate: 27.3%
Precision: 72.7%

for each feature at each node, and more – complicate the analysis. On the other hand, recent work of Biau and his many very able collaborators, shows that strong progress is being made; see Biau (2010), Biau and Devroye (2010).

Thus, it is known that some simple versions of RF are not Bayes consistent. For example, splitting to purity, such that each terminal node has only subjects of the same group, is not universally Bayes consistent. A practical message here is that terminal node sizes should be sufficiently large, and generally increase as the dataset increases. The code for Random Forests and Random Jungles allows this choice to be made by the user.

In the other direction, Random Forests can be understood as a layered nearest neighbor (LNN) scheme; see DGL (problem 11.6), as well as Lin and

Jeon (2006). In this view LNN is now known to be asymptotically optimal in the pth-mean, under mild regularity conditions. This is not the same as being Bayes consistent, let alone universally Bayes consistent (that is, Bayes consistent for all possible datasets). However, it is strongly suggestive of the strength of Random Forests.

As a practical matter, RF will function very nicely on huge datasets and enormous features lists: for example, several thousand cases and controls, and 800K SNP values for each subject. Without putting too fine a point on it, RF will usually find the signal in the data if it is there in the first place. But some other machine could do as well or better, given sufficient time and energy.

As another practical matter, RF does a routinely good job of finding the most important features in the full list. Here again no assertion of optimality is made, and multiple, distinct short lists could provide basically the same level of predictive accuracy; see Chapter 9. Yet given a plausible short list of features we can turn to other machines, ones that afford interpretability. Logistic regression applied after application of RF is one serviceable strategy. To make the claim that the predictive error has not drifted greatly when moving from RF and the full list of features to LR and a small list, it is crucial that we compare error rates. This is covered in detail in Chapter 11.

We finally comment on one other property of Random Forests. RF has the capacity to rapidly and easily generate trees, error analysis, variable importances, multidimensional scaling, and one other property: the ability to do all these tasks in the presence of missing data, but we do not take up this issue here.

Notes

(1) Random Forests has undergone several incarnations and is freely available in the R library.

    (a) A starting point is Leo Breiman's still-maintained site: www.stat. berkeley.edu/~breiman/RandomForests/.

    (b) A newer, faster version is Random Jungles, written by Daniel Schwarz, which implements several methods for feature selection and variable importance evaluations. For more on RJ see: http://randomjungle.com. And still more detail is given in Schwarz et al. (2010).

(c) The method of Conditional Inference Forests (CIF), was introduced by Carolin Strobl and her coworkers (2007, 2008). This is an important statistical innovation introduced at the node-splitting level, and often gives much better feature selection than, for example, the Gini method in RF.

(d) The key idea of random sampling from the list of features was introduced by Ho (1998).

(e) A nice series of recent lectures on RF and related methods can be found at: http://videolectures.net/sip08_biau_corfao/.

(2) We note that it would be hard to see any benefit in doing an unmodified boot draw from the feature list, doing draws with replacement. This would result in repetitions of the same features in the subset. On the other hand, if we duplicate features and rename them, say as Feature 1, Feature 2, Feature 3, etc., then seeing how often any of these were selected in any trees would provide information about the efficiency of the feature sampling. On average each of these three features should appear the same fraction of time, if the feature sampling was selecting uniformly from the entire feature list. In a very long list this question becomes more important. Thus, in a set of 500K SNPs we would want all SNPs to be considered for selection in building trees at the same rate, and exact copies of any SNPs should be in, or out, of trees at the same rate for that SNP. Getting to uniformity might require much processing time, but computational clusters and other hardware advances make this steadily less of a problem.

(3) The mathematics here is not exactly easy, but isn't that hard either. The collection of all *proximities* between any two subjects, prox(m, k) say, forms a square $N{\times}N$ matrix, where N is the sample size. With a little work it can be shown that the matrix is symmetric, positive definite, and bounded above by 1, having all diagonal elements equal to 1. It follows that the values $d(m, k) = 1-$ prox(m, k) are squared distances in a Euclidean space of dimension not greater than N; see Cox and Cox (2001). The collection of squared distances is then subject to additional transformations, and ultimately to an often-huge dimensional reduction, this using methods very similar to principal components.

Part III

Analysis fundamentals

Merely two variables

How wonderful that we have met with a paradox. Now we have some hope of making progress.

Niels Bohr

8.1 Introduction

Correlations are basic for statistical understanding. In this chapter we discuss several important examples of correlations, and what they can and cannot do. In Chapter 9 we take up more complex issues, those involving correlations and associations among several variables. We will find that statistical learning machines are an excellent environment in which to learn about connections between variables, and about the strengths and limitations of correlations.

Correlations can be used to estimate the strength of a linear relationship between two continuous variables. There are three ideas here that are central: correlations quantify *linear* relationships, they do so with only *two* variables, and the two variables are at least roughly continuous (like rainfall or temperature). If the relationship between the variables is almost linear, and we don't mind restricting ourselves to those two variables, then the prediction problem has at least one familiar solution: linear regression (see Note 1). Usually the relationship between two variables is not linear. Despite this, the relationship could still be strong, and a correlation analysis could be misleading. A statistical learning machine approach may be more likely to uncover the relationship. As a prelude to later results we show this by applying a binary decision tree to one of the examples in this chapter.

8.2 Understanding correlations

Let's start with this:

Example 8.1 Linear relationship

Height and weight were measured for 647 patients. The measurements are plotted in Figure 8.1, with weight, W (in kgs), on the vertical axis and height, H (in cms), on the horizontal axis.

The graph shows that, for this sample, W tends to increase as H increases. The estimated correlation coefficient for this sample of patients is 0.77, indicating a fairly strong linear relationship. The p-value for this mini-analysis is less than 0.0001, and so is highly significant. We would get the same correlation coefficient if we had plotted the data with W on the horizontal axis and H on the vertical, or the other way around, because correlations are symmetric. We can be fairly confident that either variable could be used as a good predictor of the other. A change in height would be expected to be associated with a proportional change in weight. The amount of change is proportional to the correlation coefficient. ◀

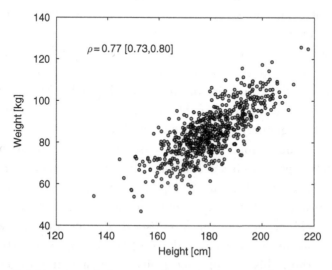

Figure 8.1   Height and weight for 647 patients. Strong correlation is present, $\rho = 0.77$ with 95% confidence interval [0.73, 0.80].

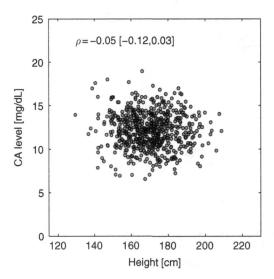

Figure 8.2   Calcium blood levels in 616 patients, plotted against height. Little correlation is present, $\rho = -0.05$, with 95% confidence interval $[-0.12, 0.03]$.

Example 8.2 No linear relationship

The level of calcium in a blood sample was also measured for 616 of the patients in Example 8.1. Figure 8.2 shows calcium, CA, plotted on the vertical axis and height, H, on the horizontal axis.

The plot shows that calcium level does not seem to depend very much on height. The estimated correlation coefficient for this pair of variables is -0.05 and hence very close to zero (the p-value is 0.26, so the estimated correlation is not considered significantly different from zero). We would probably not choose height on its own as a predictor of calcium level (or use calcium to predict height). However, it is possible that when height is combined with some other feature, then it might play a role in predicting calcium. ◀

8.3 Hazards of correlations

Here are three examples of how correlations can mislead.

Example 8.3 Outliers and linear relationships

Figure 8.3 shows data such that the main body of the data has virtually no linear relationship, yet the official, calculated correlation is very high, equal

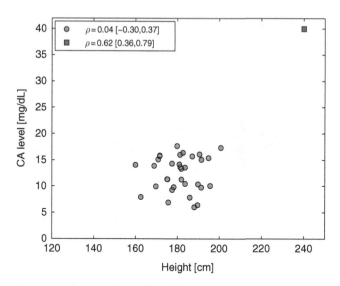

Figure 8.3   The main body of this calcium/height plot shows little correlation, $\rho = 0.04$ with 95% confidence interval [–0.30, 0.37]. Adding a single outlier at the upper right changes everything, or so it seems, with $\rho = 0.62$ and a 95% confidence interval [0.36, 0.79].

to 0.62 (the p-value is 0.01). The single data point in the upper right corner seems to be driving the correlation higher, since leaving the point out of the analysis gives a correlation of 0.04. Before casting out this data point we are obligated to ask ourselves these questions:

(1) Is this extreme data point representative of some biological process of merit? Is there a mix of different processes that might be responsible for this outlier?
(2) Are occasional extreme values typical of this process?

If the answer to either of these questions is *yes*, or if the answer is *not sure*, then the data point cannot be omitted. Only knowledge of the subject matter, and sometimes more targeted data-gathering, can resolve these questions. This decision should not be made for purely statistical reasons alone. ◀

Example 8.4 Another outlier and linear relationship
Here is the reverse situation, shown in Figure 8.4. In this example, nearly all the data have a linear structure, indicating that the correlation should be strongly positive: leaving the single data point out of the analysis gives a

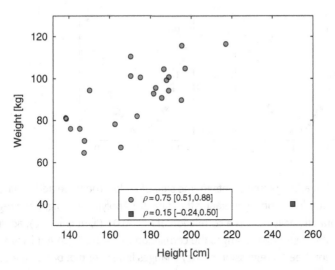

Figure 8.4   Height and weight was once strongly related, but now? The main body of the data shows a strong correlation, $\rho = 0.75$, with 95% confidence interval [0.51, 0.88]. But adding a single outlier at the lower right returns a correlation of basically zero, $\rho = 0.15$, with 95% confidence interval [–0.24, 0.50].

correlation of 0.75. However, the extreme point is masking this relationship, driving the correlation towards zero, and it is equal to 0.15. Note that the height value is unusual, as is weight, but separately each is still within the realm of the possible. However, when taken *together* it becomes clear that this data point is an outlier as it does not conform to the global pattern of the data. Whenever possible, you should always plot your data when doing correlations. See Note 2. ◀

This next example is quite important for understanding correlations and nonlinear relationships.

Example 8.5 Strong relationship but it's not linear
Consider the plot in Figure 8.5(a). Now the estimated correlation between X and Y is virtually zero, estimated at –0.01, yet the data points are clearly related. Why is the correlation coefficient so ineffective here? The answer is that any correlation only estimates the strength of a *linear* relationship. A correlation may or may not be any good at uncovering a nonlinear

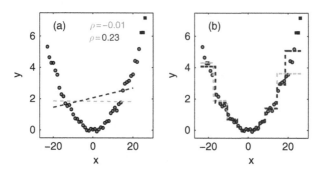

Figure 8.5.   The effect of adding three points to one side of a plot. The three additional points are from the quadratic curve generating the data. (a) Applying a straight-line regression to the data originally returns a correlation of $\rho = -0.01$ (light gray line); adding three points in the upper right changes the correlation to $\rho = 0.23$. (b) Applying a single classification tree (in regression mode) changes little over that part of the data not containing the added points, and then nicely takes the three points into account when added.

relationship, even if that alternative relationship is very strong. In this case the Xs and Ys are related (by design) as a quadratic function, $Y = X^2$.

Note also in this figure that three extra data points (squares on the upper right arm of the curve) sharply shift the correlation, and it's now 0.23 when those points are included. This seems unreasonable, since we've just added (sampled) a few more points on the same curve. Sampling a few more points on the left arm of the plot would likely return the correlation to nearly zero. The added points on the right act as if they are outliers, but in fact they are helping to refine the shape of the curve, rather than obscure the true relationship in the data.

Next, note that if we were to limit out attention to the left side of the plot, the data could be fairly well represented by a straight line (sloping downward). Similarly, if we only look at the right we could fit the data with a straight line, but sloped in the opposite direction from that on the left. This shows the distinction between looking at local versus global views of the data. The average of the two lines, in some sense, is the "correct" global line, the one that has zero slope. But does this averaging tell us about the essential predictive value of the data, given that it misses the true shape of the curve? How can we make a good prediction in this case? We could propose some function of the data that, by inspection, seems plausible: squaring the Xs, or maybe taking logarithms of the Xs – but now see the next example. ◀

The problem just discussed in Example 8.5 is important and has its own statistical literature: see Note 3.

Example 8.6 Getting the right curve

In the last example we found that a correlation approach, and a straight line, didn't fit the data very well, and tended to get confused by valid data points. We could have looked at the data plot and decided to fit a quadratic curve. This would have worked nicely here, but it would require that we guess the proper curve in light of the data. Often this works well, but in large datasets it can be hard to look over many plots and make this determination, one at a time.

To make the point that a statistical learning machine approach can sharply improve on a linear regression approach, in Figure 8.5(b) we have plotted the result of a single regression tree; see Chapter 6. This is a primitive prediction method but does well enough here. The regression tree produces a stair–step output. There are two trees and therefore two predictions for the data: the solid dots predict Y when the three "outliers" are not included, and the shaded dots predict Y when the three data points are included.

Within each segment of the data, we average the values of Y and draw a horizontal line in that segment at that average value. This is the prediction for the data in that segment. On the left-hand side of the plot, in the region near $X = -20$, the tree is estimating the Y value to be about 4, when using the solid dots *or* the shaded dots. On the right-hand side, when X is near $+20$, the shaded dots predict Y is equal to 3.5, approximately. When the extra points are included, the solid dots revise the prediction to about Y equal to 5. Finally note that most of the predictions are changed very little when the prediction is being done away from the extra points: the prediction is locally stable. This stability is good, since prediction on the right arm of the data shouldn't dramatically influence the prediction for the left arm. ◀

8.4 Correlations big and small

Correlations can appear and disappear, depending on the local nature of the data.

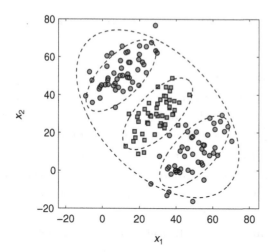

Figure 8.6   The data arises in three parts, within each of which the correlation is strongly positive. However, considered as a group the data show strong negative correlation. Strata, within-clinics, subset data need not show any obvious functional relation to pooled data: correlations don't add.

Example 8.7a Subsets of data can behave differently from the whole

We pursue this subject of local versus global. Biological datasets typically are not homogeneous, in the sense that subsets, slices, or parts of the whole, often do not look like the pooled data. In Figure 8.6 we have three clouds of data.

Taken separately they yield strong positive correlations. Taken as a whole, the general trend becomes negative, from the upper left of the plot down to the lower right. The correlation for the entire data is different from correlations for the three segments of the data, and is in the reverse direction. To make the example more compelling, suppose the data represent success rates for individual surgeons over a period of several years, plotted as a function of the total number of procedures each surgeon performed. Perhaps the three groups were collected under somewhat different research protocols, or at clinics with not-so-subtle differences in patient populations, or perhaps there are hidden, unmeasured biological processes that are causing these groups to separate. Patients at Clinic A could generally be sicker than those at Clinic B, or the surgeons at Clinic B performed the transplants under a more refined patient selection scheme. It is important in the analysis to take these additional features into account. But the context is important: within each clinic the success rate *is* positively related to the total number of procedures each surgeon performs, and this is important information. Pooling the data is an averaging that obscures this conclusion, even if we don't understand what separates the clinic results. One data analysis moral here is that correlations don't add, and unmeasured features of the data can and perhaps should sharply perturb our conclusions. But, in a large and complex dataset we may have no clue as to the number and natures of hidden variables. See Note 4. ◀

Example 8.7b Looking at subsets can induce correlation

We have just seen how pooling data can obscure or derail a relationship that exists for subsets of the data. In this example we see that a correlation and apparent structure for a subset can be an artifact of the way we create the subset. That is, starting from a data cloud with zero correlation, we can force the subset to be correlated in whatever direction we choose. Alternatively, the subsets can be driven by valid, underlying science. For this start with Figure 8.7.

We use the cholesterol data introduced in Chapter 4. The plot in Figure 8.7 shows the two cholesterol measures HDL and LDL for each of 200 patients.

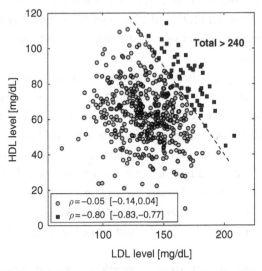

Figure 8.7   The data is uncorrelated considered as a whole, but pieces of the data need not be. There is no correlation of the data considered as a single group, but looking at just those patients with high total cholesterol shows a strong negative relationship. In this important subset of at-risk patients does this have clinical meaning?

The correlation for all patients is basically zero, equal to −0.05. The researcher is interested in whether a combined measurement of the two cholesterol values could be predictive of disease. She subsets the data to those patients having HDL + LDL above a clinically determined threshold value equal to 240, and then considers these patients to have elevated risk. Further study of these at-risk patients proceeds, and now the researcher observes that in this population HDL and LDL are strong negatively correlated, with the estimated correlation equal to −0.80.

Being a careful analyst she immediately realizes that (probably) no new science has been uncovered in this subset analysis. She is aware that this correlation was induced, since the subset does not include patients with low HDL and LDL. The moral is that it is hazardous to infer correlation from pairs of variables that were themselves used in defining the subset. Of course, this subset is still medically important since the usual definition of total cholesterol is HDL plus LDL (plus a triglyceride term; see Note 1 in Chapter 4), so that adding HDL and LDL together generates a valid tool for locating patients at risk.

She next proceeds to look at those patients having another risk factor related to cholesterol, those for whom HDL is less than 40. For this group she finds no correlation between HDL and LDL, and the subset has essentially zero correlation. Again, the analysis is statistically valid, but (probably) doesn't yield new science.

Leaving aside the problem of how subgroups may or may not reflect group structure, she now has defined two, distinct at-risk populations, those patients with high total cholesterol, HDL + LDL more than 240, and those with low HDL. Each group represents patients with well-studied clinical problems. Is it possible, she asks, to more reliably classify patients using both of these risk factors? This is different from the regression-style prediction problem in Example 8.6 above. It also presents a challenge in classifying at-risk patients, since the at-risk region of the data is wedge-shaped and not separated by a single, easy-to-describe, straight-line boundary. ◀

Summarizing so far, we suggest using correlations under these conditions: (a) you are able to look at your data in a plot, or at least able to look at several small random subsamples of the data; (b) there are no outliers, or you have examined the unusual points and made some scientific decision about their inclusion or exclusion; (c) it appears that a linear relation will adequately characterize the data; and (d) there are no problems with local vs. global grouping effects, such as we saw in Example 8.7a, or else your subsequent analyses take the grouping into account.

In Chapter 9 we study data for which we may not have the luxury of looking at all possible plots, or for which strong linear relationships may exist but they don't capture the true structure of the data, and for which local behavior has to take precedence over global.

Let's end this chapter with another look at the two datasets above, those having outliers. For each we apply a single decision tree, used in regression mode.

In Figure 8.8, a single tree meanders through the body of the data but also passes through the "outlier" in the upper right. In Figure 8.9 we see that the outlier on the lower right is correctly predicted, even though this point may not be valid scientifically. On the other hand, the main body of the data isn't that well covered by the tree prediction: the line segment predictions don't

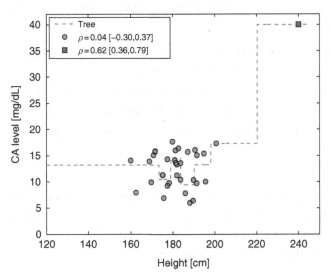

Figure 8.8   A single tree is applied to data, the main body of which does not contain a strong signal, with a correlation close to zero. But the tree does get, once more, the single outlier. In this case meandering through the central portion of the data is not necessarily a mistake, but a forest approach would likely smooth the central prediction. However, passing through the single extreme point is probably misleading, unless the underlying science says otherwise.

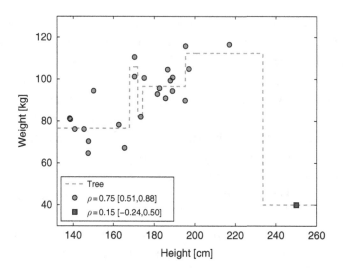

Figure 8.9   A single decision tree nails the "outlier" on the lower right, but meanders through the main body of the data. The central portion of the data does contain a signal, as the correlation is strong and the data there looks linear, but the tree seems uncertain. Reducing the terminal node size of the single tree, or using a forest of trees might help; see Chapter 7.

move smoothly upward from left to right as we might expect given the strong correlation of this central part of the data.

That is, single trees may not work automatically well with relatively small amounts of data. Another way to state this result is by reference to Section 2.11: the rate of convergence to optimality may be rather slow for single trees.

Notes

(1) To understand what the correlation represents we need to start with its definition. Assume that Y and X are related by the linear equation $Y = a + bX +$ error for some constants a and b.

Then the correlation is given by

$$\rho = b \times \frac{\sigma_X}{\sigma_Y},$$

where

b = slope of the linear regression line $Y = a + bX$
a = intercept of the line with the Y-axis

σ_Y = standard deviation of the distribution for Y

σ_X = standard deviation of the distribution for X.

When Y and X are rescaled so that both have standard deviation equal to one, we find that $\rho = b$, which emphasizes the connection between correlation and that term in the equation above for Y. In the regression analysis framework, given the data we replace the mathematical constants above with estimated values.

(2) Addressing the problem of unusual observations has two parts. First, we need to devise a method for uncovering observations that markedly stand out from the others, and then second, settle upon a method for dealing with the unusual observations. As we saw in Examples 8.3 and 8.4, finding an observation that sticks out requires looking at each variable separately and the variables together. However we choose to resolve this first problem – of declaring something unusual – we still need to deal with the second problem: what to do when an outlier is detected. Deleting a data point is not something we recommend generally, but down-weighting or reducing the impact of the data point on the subsequent analysis is one alternative. Or we can consider an analysis in which the data point is included, then one in which it isn't included, and compare the results. This is an example of studying the robustness of the inference, which we strongly recommend; see, for example, Spiegelhalter and Marshall (2006). We could also use alternative definitions for correlations. That is, methods have been proposed that are less sensitive to outliers, but they are also less familiar so that it can be difficult to grasp what they mean precisely in a practical sense. See for example:

http://www.stat.ubc.ca/~ruben/website/chilsonthesis.pdf.

Also Alqallaf *et al.* (2002), Hardin *et al.* (2007). A central point to keep in mind, no matter how you choose to thread a path through these data analysis choices, is this: fully declare the method by which any data point is considered to be unusual (an outlier) and disclose the method used to treat that data point.

(3) It is easy to construct examples of a distribution for a random variable X and then define a pair (X, Y) for $Y = X^2$ such that: $cor(X^m, Y^n) = 0$, for

every positive odd integer *m* and any positive integer *n*. Indeed, simply let X have any distribution symmetric around $X = 0$; see Mukhopadhyay (2009), as well as Hamedani and Volkmer (2009).

(4) This slippery problem is so recurrent that it has its own name: *Simpson's paradox*. As with many paradoxes, it arises when one assumption or another has been overlooked or in which the outcome measure is itself ambiguous. In this case the problem is that the subgroups don't reflect the behavior of the pooled data. Here the misleading assumption is that a single number, the pooled correlation, can speak for the entire dataset, when it is better represented in terms of two or more correlations, a pooled value and separate values for the subgroups. If the subsections of the data all show similar behavior then it is possible to borrow strength from the subsections, to create a more efficient single summary. This forms the statistical subject of *analysis of covariance* and *multilevel models*: see, for example, Twisk (2006).

9

More than two variables

... beware of mathematicians, and all those who make empty prophecies. The danger already exists that the mathematicians have made a covenant with the devil to darken the spirit and to confine man in the bonds of Hell.

St. Augustine

9.1 Introduction

Even when we understand the benefits and hazards of correlations among pairs of variables we are not guaranteed solid footing when it comes to understanding relationships among slightly more involved sets of variables. Consider a problem involving just three variables, such as studying the connection between the features X, Y, and the outcome variable Z. Such data is the primary recurrent example studied in this chapter. Simple correlations do not easily deal with this situation since sets of features can act in highly coordinated but not obvious ways. The error often made here is assuming that such coordination within three (or more) features can be described using a single summary statistic. Moreover, such entangled data occurs frequently in biology and clinical medicine, and complex versions of this problem can involve hundreds or thousands of such interacting features. This is especially true for broad-scale -omics data, which includes proteomics, genomics, and other newer biological collections that continue to be organized. Statistical learning machines are well suited to dealing with these coordination problems, and we document their utility by discussing examples of these problems. We conclude with a problem related to lists of predictive variables: how to join multiple lists together into a single, best list.

9.2 Tiny problems, large consequences

The following two examples have all the relevant features understood and measured – nothing is hidden. Yet the analysis in each case is not obvious and is therefore troubling. For this reason they are deeply instructive (or, should be). The problems relate to the biomechanics of walking, and blood flow.

Example 9.1 One variable is not enough

A clinician is studying spinal curvature. A normal spine appears straight when a patient is observed from the back. Pathologic spinal curvature, or scoliosis, is present when the spine does not appear straight from the back. The clinician makes rigorous and time-consuming measurements of angles along the spine as deviations from one vertebra to the next or the true vertical. She also measures the lengths of patients' legs, hoping that these length measurements can be used to predict curvature and reduce the need to make painstaking angle measurements in the future. She finds, not surprisingly, that the right leg length is highly correlated with the left leg length. She has heard that when two variables are highly correlated, one of them can (should!) be omitted from the analysis. However, the right leg length is not at all correlated with the measurement of curvature, and neither is the left leg length. She knows that tall people as well as short people can have curved spines, so it isn't the actual length that would be predictive of curvature. Sometimes spinal curvature is associated with differences in leg lengths. The clinician computes the right leg length minus the left leg length, and then calculates the correlation coefficient of that with spinal curvature. The *difference* in leg length is highly correlated with spinal curvature! Both variables were needed to be able to predict spinal curvature. Also, it is possible to have legs the same length, but still have either zero or some spinal curvature. These patients will need a different set of features; see Note 1. ◀

Another way of describing the problem just discussed is that there are hazards when deleting features as predictors if they are either pairwise correlated with each other, or, are each separately uncorrelated with some outcome variable. In fact, the features might individually have a profoundly negative effect on the health of the organism (including lethality), but jointly might be essential to good functioning. In genetics this phenomenon has its own name, *epistasis*; see Note 2.

Let's further examine this coordinated activity of features, by looking at the same pair of features across a big evolutionary range, and within an organism.

Example 9.2 Two variables and the importance of context

The fact that variables can together be useful when the value of each by itself is not, is a quite pervasive occurrence in biological data. Consider the problem of monitoring cardiac functioning, *CF*, for an organism where we measure the amount of blood going into the heart, *A*, and the amount of blood leaving the heart, *B*. It is well known that the total amount of blood entering, *A*, should be approximately equal to the amount, *B*, leaving the heart, under the premise that the circulation and the cardiac system is functionally normally. It is also the case that *A* and *B* are highly correlated, except under extreme deviations from cardiac sufficiency. And it is known that the absolute amounts of blood entering the heart, or leaving the heart, can both have quite wide ranges, so that high values of *A* and high values of *B* (or relatively low values for both) may be perfectly normal and not point to any cardiac problems. Predicting normal *CF* for the system then is, to a good approximation, done using the *ratio* of the two volumes (per minute, say): $CF = A / B$. See Note 3.

If the whale, human, or mouse suffers some catastrophic interruption in normal blood flow (an artery is cut, or return flow is impeded by a clot) then there would be a sharp imbalance in the input/output ratio: *CF* would move sharply away from $CF = 1$, and left unattended this could be lethal. Consider next the situation where both output and input are unusually low (for that organism). This is typical of the clinical condition of cardiac insufficiency. In this case the ratio *CF* could still be close to one, so that the ratio by itself would not be especially predictive of a clinical problem. The time course for this problem could also be much longer, months or years long for a human. Thus a short-term, highly lethal event could be detected by the *CF* ratio departing from one, and a long-term, possibly lethal event not detected by any departure of the *CF* ratio from one.

This discussion for humans applies just as well to whales and mice, and it does so for these organisms under most conditions of activity: a human running up a flight of stairs or standing still to adjust her iPod; a mouse on a treadmill or sound asleep; a whale swimming quietly or swimming fast to avoid a cruise ship loaded with a group of sympathetic but over-eager sightseers, and then swimming quietly again. All three organisms change their levels of A and B markedly (up or down) and in order to maintain normal cardiac function. In fact, normal $CF = 1$ is closely maintained for these three diverse organisms with each having very different total blood volumes, and with very distinct normal heart pumping rates. This model therefore applies over a wide range of species, with large evolutionary separations, and at most points of time within the separate lives of the individuals. However, $CF = 1$ does not by itself define healthy cardiac function: the ratio is diagnostic for some events, and not others. ◀

We have seen that correlations among the features, and between the features and the outcome variable, can be deceptive as well as informative. Let's see if a more statistically rigorous approach can disentangle some of these slippery aspects of features and outcomes.

9.3 Mathematics to the rescue?

Adding more techniques to a project may or may not be productive.

Example 9.3 Maybe we just need more excellent mathematics
In this example the correlations of each of the features with the outcome are not zero, yet there is still paradoxical behavior. Somewhat buried in their magisterial three-volume work, Kendall and Stuart (1979, p. 350) present a very accessible example. It is the problem of estimating Y = crop yield (in cwt per acre), using the features R = total rainfall (in inches), and T = cumulative temperature (in deg F). We write cor(Y, R) for the correlation between crop yield and rainfall, cor(Y, T) for the correlation between crop yield and temperature, and cor(R, T) for the correlation between rainfall and temperature. Then the starting data is:

$$\text{mean}(Y) = 28.02, \quad \text{mean}(R) = 4.91, \quad \text{mean}(T) = 594,$$
$$\text{var}(Y) = 4.42, \quad \text{var}(R) = 1.10, \quad \text{var}(T) = 85, \tag{9.1}$$
$$\text{cor}(Y, R) = +0.80 \quad \text{cor}(Y, T) = -0.40, \quad \text{cor}(R, T) = -0.56.$$

Our challenge here is to both predict crop yield, from rainfall and temperature, and perhaps more importantly, to better understand the connection between crop yield and these two predictors. From the data above we see that crop yield is positively related to rainfall, since cor(Y, R) = +0.80, but it is negatively related to temperature, since cor(Y, T) = −0.40. This reversal of correlations seems to track well with the negative correlation between temperature and rainfall, as cor(R, T) = −0.56. On the other hand, the prediction equation we obtain from simple linear regression takes the form:

$$Y = 9.311 + 3.37 \times R + 0.0036 \times T \qquad (9.2)$$

(where we have written the equation with the variables each centered to have mean zero). In this equation we see that, *if we hold rainfall constant*, crop yield is *positively* related to temperature, since the coefficient for T is 0.0036 > 0.

One way to understand the processes here is to calculate *partial correlations*. Mathematically, it tells us about the (linear) relationship between two variables, *given* that the third (or, all the others) is being held constant; see Note 4.

In this case the partial correlation of yield with respect to temperature, cor $(Y$ and T, given $R)$ = 0.097, is positive, telling us that crop yield increases as does temperature, *given a fixed value of rainfall*. A similar calculation reveals that:

$$\text{cor}(Y \text{ and } R, \text{ given } T) = 0.759$$
$$\text{cor}(R \text{ and } T, \text{ given } Y) = -0.436, \qquad (9.3)$$

showing that crop yield rises as does rainfall at constant temperature, but that temperature and rainfall are negatively related, *conditional on a given crop yield.*◀

The challenge posed by this example, and others like it, is this: can we put these differing relationships, these differing correlation results, into some single, consistent framework? That is, since cor$(Y$ and T, given $R)$ = 0.097, is crop yield *positively* related to rainfall? Or, since cor(Y, T) =−0.40, is it *negatively* related? How can it be both?

The paradox here does have a resolution: these conflicted correlations are addressing different questions. A less obscure, more mathematical reply is this: the answer depends on the context of the question, and it may be better to have good questions than to insist on a single right answer. This (hardly original) insight will appear frequently in our discussion of statistical learning. The functional, apparent scientific connection between sets of predictors and an outcome variable can change dramatically depending on the sets of predictors under study. The mathematics of regression, and functional relationships generally, is this: how a predictor appears in relation to an outcome is a function of the other predictors in the model – the local network – of the given predictor. There is no mathematical conflict here and unfortunately also no general mathematical scheme by which a single universal and consistent reply is possible to this problem of conflicted correlations.

9.4 Good models need not be unique

The problem of finding good models is too often based on the assumption that the data can be decisive about the goodness of any single model. This is usually *not* the case, and this issue is quite important for our understanding of statistical learning machines and data analysis generally.

Example 9.4 Multiple models can be equally good
Consider predicting beer consumption, $Y = \log$(beer consumption in barrels), during the interwar years 1920–1939 in the UK; see Kendall (1980).

$$A = \log(\text{real income}),$$
$$B = \log(\text{retail price}),$$
$$C = \log(\text{cost} - \text{of} - \text{living index}), \qquad (9.4)$$
$$D = \log(\text{specific gravity of beer}),$$
$$E = \log(\text{time}).$$

The author found (in 1945) that the predictors $\{A, B, C, D, E\}$ were highly correlated among themselves (both positively and negatively so), and reported a range of correlations of the predictors with the outcome variable (again positive and negative). Of most interest to us is a set of regression equations he derived:

Model 1 : $Y = 0.282 \times A - 0.309 \times B + 0.978 \times C + 0.123 \times D - 0.231 \times E$
$$R^2 = 0.9896$$

Model 2 : $Y = 1.251 \times C + 0.549 \times D + 0.686 \times E$
$$R^2 = 0.9676$$

Model 3 : $Y = -0.021 \times A - 0.472 \times B + 1.097 \times C$
$$R^2 = 0.9808.$$
$$(9.5)$$

In describing the predictive accuracy of these three models we quoted above the value for R^2, the *coefficient of determination*; see Note 5.

As a first observation we see that all the models do really well, and are indeed indistinguishable, since $R^2 \approx 1$ in all cases. The second point is that the models are themselves distinguishable, especially Models 2 and 3, which overlap only slightly in the use of the predictors: $\{C, D, E\}$ for Model 2, and $\{A, B, C\}$ for Model 3. The conclusion to be drawn here is: very different models can have very similar predictive accuracy. ◄

The conclusion just derived is an extremely important idea, especially in the context of machine learning models. That is, how features work together in Nature is often hidden from us, and very different sets of features (in models) can work together very well. It is often true that the features themselves are highly related, but in problems with many – possibly hundreds or thousands – of features how they collaborate, how they internally coordinate their actions, is a mystery that often requires considerable experiment and interpretation. But in a more positive direction, if something important is occurring in the data, we can expect to find it, and do so with more than one good model. Nature is often mysterious, seemingly random, but she is never malicious.

Example 9.5 Correlations don't add

Here is a less esoteric treatment of this problem of coordination among multiple features. The coefficient of determination, R^2, is not just the sum of the simple correlations across the features in the model. Indeed, it is relatively easy to construct data for predicting y from x_1 and x_2, such that $R^2 = 1$ (exactly!) yet the simple correlations $\text{cor}(y, x_1)$ and $\text{cor}(y, x_2)$ are both arbitrarily close to zero. Indeed, it is easy to arrange for one of these simple correlations to be exactly zero. The prediction equation here is not at all complex, being a linear sum of x_1 and x_2: $y = ax_1 + bx_2$. This counter-example is yet another version of the rule: *correlations don't add*. There is elementary geometry that is helpful for understanding this state of affairs; see, for example, Kendall (1980, chapter 7). ◄

We have been discussing how correlations can help or hinder our understanding of the problem of estimating an outcome, such as spinal curvature. The problem of using any single measure for evaluating the connection between a feature and the outcome appears in very simple problems as we have seen. Here is one that is supremely simple and a shock to the system of even the most battle-hardened data analyst.

Example 9.6 Role reversals for just three binary variables

DGL (theorem 32.2) and Toussaint (1971) consider the following example. It makes many of the same points as above in our discussion of regression problems, but now in the setting of decision rules. In this case the probabilities of all the values and outcomes for every feature are completely known. We assume an outcome y is binary, and we have a decision problem, using any combinations of three features, $\{x_1, x_2, x_3\}$. Each of the xs is also binary, and we ask for the best possible (smallest) error values in using any subset of the predictors; see Chapter 11 for more on error analysis and also Section 2.11 earlier. Then there exists a probability distribution for y and the xs such that the best possible decisions have these Bayes error values, L:

$$
\begin{aligned}
&L(x_1) < L(x_2) < L(x_3), \\
&L(x_1, x_2) > L(x_1, x_3) > L(x_2, x_3).
\end{aligned}
\tag{9.6}
$$

See Note 6 for the specific probabilities behind this model, and the associated calculations.

Here's what this means: having the lowest Bayes error values for single predictors is x_1, followed by x_2 and yet the best pair of predictors is $\{x_2, x_3\}$. Moreover, while the weakest *single* predictors are x_2 and x_3, the best *pair* of predictors are exactly these, $\{x_1, x_2\}$. It is also interesting to observe the equivocal, shifting role played by x_2: (a) it is an intermediate individual predictor, and (b) it interacts nicely with x_3 to yield the best predictive pair, but (c) it drags down the predictive strength of x_1, the best single predictor; and finally there is this (d) the best predictor pair does not contain the best single predictor.

Another aspect of this example is this: given the outcome y (group membership, $y = 0$ or 1, say) the three features are statistically independent. This means that correlations among the features are not sufficient to explain the role reversals of the example: within each of the two groups the features are statistically independent.

A further comment about this situation. In Elashoff *et al.* (1967), it is shown that for binary features, having a positive correlation among pairs can *increase* the predictive power of the model and *lower* the optimal error rate, the Bayes error. This remark applies therefore to SNPs and any other binary genetic marker predictors: SNPs in strong correlation with each other – or in linkage disequilibrium blocks – can be *more* predictive than those not so correlated. It should not be automatic that they be filtered or discarded. ◀

9.5 Contexts and coefficients

Another important lesson here is this: exactly how a feature makes an appearance in any model can change dramatically across a set of equally good models. Thus, in Model 1 we find the coefficient for A is positive (= +0.282), in Model 2 the coefficient is (effectively) zero, while in Model 3 it is negative (= −0.021). Which is to say that the influence of a predictor in a single model is highly dependent on the other predictors present in the model. How a predictor appears in a model is context-dependent. Acting as if a single best model exists, or a single scheme by which a feature makes a contribution, is largely a convenience for the data analyst. Biologically it may not be sensible to assume a single such model exists, or a single mechanism for each feature.

This lack of a single good model, or more correctly the unitary assumption that such a perfect solitary model exists, has the potential for highly conflicted scientific reporting. Thus, an investigator having collected data for Model 1 at some considerable time and expense (perhaps) could wish to claim that feature A is positively correlated with the outcome Y, given constant values for the other predictors, while an investigator driven by Model 2 could claim that feature A has no usefulness for predicting outcome, while the investigator behind Model 3 could claim that both the other two investigators are quite mistaken, and in fact A is negatively related to the outcome. Indeed, it is possible that no more data and no additional analysis are required to sort out these sharply differing outcomes – *they can all be correct*, in the contexts in which the claims are made. See Note 7.

A further complicating fact is this: within the confines of a single (linear or logistic) model, it is still mathematically correct to view A, for example, as making a positive contribution to the overall prediction in the context of Model 1. It is also correct to claim that A makes a negative contribution, within the prediction afforded by Model 2. That is, the contribution for each need not be constant across multiple contexts (models), but it is valid to report a positive (negative, or null) contribution to a single model.

Kendall (1980) nicely summarizes the situation by stating that: *It is the equation as a whole, not the coefficients of individual terms, which is important* (italics in the original). Our point is that in the case of statistical learning machines, where single, easily understood prediction equations for outcomes may not be visible (or even part of the machine's design), this observation about the appearance of predictors is still in force, when we seek to find a simplifying model, such as a linear or logistic regression model; see Chapter 5.

Example 9.7 Very different-looking equations but acting the same
Here is another example of how very different-looking equations can have very similar predictions, this time using nonlinear models. Figure 9.1 shows plots of two functions that are mathematically distinct, yet nearly identical over the range of the data collected.

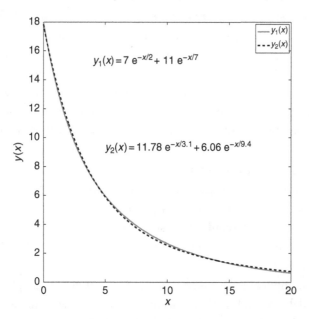

$$y_1(x) = 7\,e^{-x/2} + 11\,e^{-x/7}$$

$$y_2(x) = 11.78\,e^{-x/3.1} + 6.06\,e^{-x/9.4}$$

Figure 9.1   Two curves, with very different-looking equations, but essentially identical plots over the displayed range. What does this mean for data collection? For declaring one model better than another?

Such differences that aren't really differences are common in nonlinear modeling. We expect to see this, especially in statistical learning machine schemes. The equations for these models, and the mathematics at work here, are given in Note 8. Moreover, we are likely to find that collecting more data may not change our conclusions significantly, in that over the range of data, X, collected the two curves will remain effectively distinct, as mathematical or statistical objects, and not separable in terms of their ability to fit the data. In such cases, making strong claims for one model or another, in terms of coefficient signs or sizes, or in terms of predictive accuracy, is misguided. ◀

In view of the several examples above we assert that: if Nature has anything to say, she will do so in a variety of languages. Multiple, good models, each very different from each other, is the norm when anything interesting is occurring in the data.

9.6 Interpreting and testing coefficients in models

We have seen how unstable and possibly unhelpful individual coefficients in a model can be, especially when considered in isolation, that is, without accounting for the entanglements between one feature and all the other features. We have also seen, through our use of partial correlations, that some good interpretive sense can be derived from the model coefficients. And we've also seen that viewing all the model terms in succession, can lead to statistically incoherent statements. Thus the only firm conclusion here is that interpreting coefficients within a single model is hazardous, and we compound the statistical incoherence when we try to impose a unified understanding of a single model coefficient across several plausible models.

Attempting to resolve these conflicts while avoiding detours into incoherence is both a noble and doomed enterprise, in our opinion. But it is a large, sprawling, still-evolving object of considerable statistical study; see Note 9. The particular method under attack is that of stepwise regression. Our comments apply equally to stepwise logistic regression, and stepwise discriminant analysis. Indeed, this last, very classical method is mathematically re-expressible as a form of ordinary linear regression; see, for example, Kshirsagar (1972).

All such methods basically work this way: (1) a large model is specified, one having many features; (2) a single feature is selected from the list and its individual contribution to the full model is evaluated, using some statistical figure of merit; (3) if the statistical evaluation of that single feature shows that it contributes little to the overall model prediction, then it is deleted; (4) having deleted a feature the process is repeated, using the remaining features in the reduced model. This process continues until a small set of features is obtained such that no feature deletion can be made without a statistically significant reduction in predictive capacity. This method just described corresponds to a version of backward stepwise elimination. A forward stepwise approach starts with a single feature and adds additional terms until no change in predictive capacity is observed. Numerous subloops have been devised for both of these methods, involving the reinsertion of features into the process from among those previously deleted. The statistical figure-of-merit is often a familiar quantity, such as a t-test, and this yields a p-value, upon which the decision to delete or not is based. The multiple p-values generated this way typically have no practical statistical value, as each is computed *conditional* on all the other tests and the p-values already generated.

It is difficult to say too much that is unfairly critical of this class of methods: we strongly recommend that stepwise methods not be used unless extreme measures are taken to validate the results; see Chapter 11.

Still, it might be thought possible to mathematically adjust the tests of significance obtained by any scheme. However, to start with a model generated using a stepwise approach, and then make subtle mathematical adjustments, is a path that leads to a state of depression (at least for one of the authors) rather than to a good model. That is, the stepwise approach is not provably guaranteed to find *any* good, small model, so that a good estimate of the model it does obtain will often be much worse than the small model obtained using non-stepwise methods.

Yet, when in this process we encounter terms in the model that are statistically not different from zero, or are essentially zero on a practical basis, it stands to reason these terms could be dropped from the model with little cost in predictive accuracy, and much gain in interpretability for the smaller model so obtained. This is a seemingly sensible practice if applied to a single term in the model. It is, however, quite mistaken when applied wholesale to more than one term in the model. The technical problem is not the specifics of the test we use for, say, each of a pair of terms one after the other. The problem is, rather, that having tested one term for equality to zero, we are not statistically or mathematically free to set that term to zero and proceed to consider other terms, because testing that involves any other term assumes (usually) that all other terms are in the model. That is, each test of a single term is testing if, given that all other terms in the model are present, the term in question adds any new information (predictive power) to the model.

Consider, for example, the following often-used testing sequence. In a model with variables A, B, C, look at the model coefficient Coef_A for variable A. This means, perform the test for $\text{Coef}_A = 0$ given that $\text{Coef}_B \neq 0$, $\text{Coef}_C \neq 0$. Suppose that on the basis of this test we declare $\text{Coef}_A = 0$. Next we consider testing $\text{Coef}_B = 0$. In isolation, testing the coefficient for variable B is certainly sensible, but this test assumes that all other terms are present in the model, including A, so that the test is assuming $\text{Coef}_A \neq 0$, which we just decided was not true. The same thing happens when testing any of the coefficients in the model, one at a time. That is, a commonly used testing strategy has an internal logical conflict that can't be repaired.

More troubling still are technical results showing that if a term in the model, say, that for variable A, is not truly zero but is considered to be zero (on the basis of some t-test, for example, or experimental judgment) then the subsequent t-test for the coefficient for variable B will not have the assumed t-distribution. It can, indeed, be bimodal, having two peaks and hence not even close to a normal or t-distribution. The subsequent test for B can be arbitrarily incorrect, and this holds no matter what the sample size; for technical details see Leeb (2005), Leeb and Pötscher (2005, 2006), Kabaila and Leeb (2006). One of the main ideas in this discussion is that the large-sample approach to the correct parameter values for a smaller, correct model – after model selection is done with the data at hand – can be arbitrarily slow and far from uniform as the sample size grows.

This approach to infinity is a nontrivial consideration and is something we first mentioned in Section 2.11, in our discussion of the convergence rate to the Bayes error limit for one learning machine or another. Here it's not even true that the rate is simply slow, as it can be arbitrarily slow depending on the true model and parameter values. Rather, contrary to the study by Molinaro *et al.*

2005, it is not simply sufficient that we do repeated bootstrap sampling, say, over model selection and parameter estimation given the data. This may reduce the error involved but, finally, the process of finding and properly estimating the true smaller model is provably very hard. And closely related to this is the problem of estimating the error for the model selected; see Chapter 11.

Example 9.8 Hazards of testing one variable at a time

Using our leg length and spinal curvature problem discussed earlier we can construct an informative counter-example to the common scheme of testing one variable at a time. Thus, suppose variables A, and B, both represent slightly different measurements of right leg length, or, suppose that one of these, A, represents right leg length, while B represents some other medical value that is known to be highly correlated with right leg length. Consider a second pair of variables, C and D, of this same type, where both represent left leg length in some sense or are highly correlated. Now in a model that has variables $\{A, C, D\}$ we would find that adding variables is redundant – the coefficient would be found to be zero, for statistical purposes. We would also find that in the model $\{B, C, D\}$ the coefficient for A would be statistically zero. Therefore, if we used a "test one variable at a time" scheme we would now find that both A and B should be dropped from the final, best model. But this isn't right, since we know that the reduced model using just $\{C, D\}$ has virtually no predictive power for spinal curvature: these variables are both versions of left leg length, which is uncorrelated with spinal curvature by itself. A similar argument shows that the model $\{A, B\}$ has no predictive power, while the models $\{A, B, C\}$, $\{A, B, D\}$, $\{A, D\}$, $\{A, C\}$, $\{B, C\}$, $\{B, D\}$, all have excellent predictive power. To summarize, checking the importance of each variable one at a time and dropping as we went along would have led us to toss out an entire menagerie of good models. ◀

For the several reasons above we strongly suggest avoiding single, one-at-a-time tests for terms in the model; stepwise methods are of this type. Moreover, we have seen in Example 9.4 that multiple models can fit the data very well, with some variables having coefficients exactly zero. It would be equally incorrect, therefore, to delete every term that appeared in one of the models with a zero coefficient. In the example above we would retain only the single variable C. Since we do not have access to the data in this example, and we cannot determine whether or not the single variable C could do as well as all the others, in various groupings, this would seem to be a low percentage play, and not a recommended strategy.

We pause to consider why it is that such methods are still being widely used, as it provides insight into the use and misuse of some data-mining methods, including the ones we discuss or promote in the pages below. The principle reason appears to be the well-studied fact that the conventional statistical calculations in these schemes nearly uniformly result in optimistic outcomes, showing very high R^2 values, and very low apparent prediction error rates. The methods are not simply biased, sometimes too optimistic and sometimes too pessimistic in terms of prediction error rates or prediction accuracy, but rather are consistently too optimistic. Such apparent optimism results in data outcomes that nearly always find something of interest occurring in the data, something not pure noise and strongly predictive. Researchers naturally would like such statistical outcomes, and the statistically faulty schemes nicely cooperate. Thus, we conclude that such methods are still being used and still being widely merchandized since they fill an emotional need, not a scientific one.

Improved statistical practice, using alternative methods for calculating figures of merit such as R^2, can lead to relatively unbiased, and more trustworthy analyses. However, not often appearing in the formal studies of the breakdown and repair of these methods is a darker problem, one that is present even when we use a nearly optimal method for uncovering structure and meaning in our data. It is also a valid and important problem for statistical learning generally.

Namely, when any scheme announces that these features (this particular model, this clever construction) show great promise, we naturally try to support or understand the analytic results using our carefully acquired understanding of the subject matter itself. In our experience, however, this form of reverse engineering virtually always leads to sensible, plausible statements, such as "well, of course, these features show up as the most predictive, as they are all functions of HLA genes and these are known to be predictive of inflammation." Indeed, the more we deeply understand the subject matter, the more likely it is that nearly *any* feature set showing *any* predictive or explanative power, can be supported after the fact with plausible science.

This is not to argue for intentionally limiting our understanding of the subject matter we are trying to decode using a given statistical learning method. It does argue, instead, for considerable caution in how we justify any analytic outcome. The standard antidote for these easily generated plausibility constructions is replication of the experiment under similar or possibly carefully mutated experimental set-ups. An alternative approach to full replication begins with this, a point we have touched on earlier: for a given dataset there are usually multiple, very different-looking models that fit equally well and each of these can be expected to tell a slightly different story about the underlying mechanisms under study. Thus we can ask how the multiple models can have related or overlapping explanations, each plausible when considered separately. We consider examples of this multiple model approach in Chapter 12. In a sense to be made more precise later on, the method of Random Forests (discussed in Chapter 7) takes this multiple model approach to one logical extreme, by randomly sampling from a large space of models. Before we discuss this family of multiple model approaches, however, we need to understand the process of randomly sampling for the data itself, and why this can be so useful. This we do in Chapter 10.

Let's review some of the important conclusions from the examples just discussed, and consider further examples.

Straightforward and apparently sensible schemes for sifting through data for relationships can easily and often be in error. For the purpose of predicting Y, discarding the usefulness of both A and B if they *separately* show little relationship to Y, is quite mistaken. More broadly, we say that successful prediction is often based on how the variables connect with each other as "networked" collaborators that are jointly predictive, and indeed, truly weak predictors can be powerful especially if they are relatively uncorrelated among themselves; see Note 10.

This insight can be given a mathematical foundation that we take up in Chapter 11.

9.7 Merging models, pooling lists, ranking features

Let's suppose now that we have at least one good model for prediction, and are presented with another model or several such. Let's further assume that both models are reasonably good (low error values) and that there isn't any compelling statistical reason to distinguish the two models. That is, estimating the error value for each model (prediction engine) shows that both are pretty good (however we choose to define that for the given problem), and that we have no statistical inference argument to suggest that one is better than the other; for details on both these technical steps, see Chapter 10.

It is then likely the case that the two models reason from rather distinct lists of features: Model A, generated using some collection of learning machines, uses the features (a, b, c), while Model B, generated using some other possibly overlapping set of machines, uses the features (a, b, d, e). In this situation one list is entirely contained in the other. If there is no statistical reason to think any predictive information has been lost in reporting Model A instead of Model B, then parsimony suggests just reporting the smaller model.

A few words of caution: the reasoning just used is reminiscent of the 14th century maxim known as Occam's Razor: entities should not be multiplied without necessity. See Note 11. There are at least two problems with this approach.

First, it conflates simplicity with simple explanations: an apparently simple phenomenon may have a complex mechanism. For example, alerting the reader to Model B will point to its use of the "extra" features (d, e) beyond those appearing in Model A, and looking into the predictive capacity of those features as *biological entities*, as components in a larger and significant metabolic pathway for example, could be very instructive. Pointing to the pathway as a whole suggests a comprehensive and therefore better model.

Second, defining *simplicity* is itself complex. It is possible that quoting Occam's Razor in any argument introduces needless secondary issues and should be avoided. For example, in reporting (a, b, c) as superior to (a, b, c, d, e) we have assumed that shorter is simpler. What then to make of two lists of the form (a, b, c) and (a, d, e)? Here as elsewhere we could consider that we are really given two lists of the same features, but with different weights attached: the first list "includes" features d and e, but with reduced, indeed zero weight, while the second reduces the importance of features b and e to effectively zero. Viewing the list problem as one of *importances* leads us to the general problem of this section, that of joining or merging two lists of identical features, but where the lists give different weights to the features.

Thus suppose we are given two lists of predictive features where we order the lists according to the importances each model (each machine) assigns to the features. We make no assumptions about the merit of each such list of weights. They could in fact be generated by the same modeling scheme, the same machine, but on *different* samples from the same biological process, or from the *same* data under two bootstrap draws.

The list-merging problem as just outlined is actually the preference (or voting) problem; see Note 12. Consider, then, this situation. Using the features $\{a, b, c\}$, three machines generate a preference list, that is, an ordering of the features according to their apparent predictive power:

Machine A generates list (a, b, c)
Machine B generates list (b, c, a)
Machine C generates list (c, a, b).

Here, all three machines find predictive power in just the three features, but their code generates a ranking of the features in terms of relative predictive power, so that Machine A orders (ranks) feature a more predictive than b, and b more predictive than c.

We ask, shouldn't it be possible to come to some agreement as to the importance of these features, some super-list of preferences? Surprisingly, the answer from theory is no, and is an example of Condorcet's voting paradox dating from 1785. Here is a problem with a possible super-list. If we decide to merge the rankings by majority vote then a beats b (two of the three machines put a ahead of b), and b beats c (two of the three machines put b ahead of c), but also c beats a (two of the three machines put c ahead of a).

It gets worse. If we choose to proceed in a stepwise manner then we can consider just voting on any two of the pairs, a against b, say, and then from the winner of that vote, consider how it compares with the third feature. Under this entirely plausible scheme we will *always* find that the third feature wins. For example, comparing just a against b we find that a comes out ahead with two of the three machines (just as above). But comparing it against c we now find that c always wins (two out of the three machines). This argument is valid if we start with b against c, finding that a always wins at the second step, or starting with a against c, when b always wins at the second step.

These preference problems are troubling. They can't be fixed in general, in that some lists of preferences won't lead to the conflicts above, but many do. A more recent statement of the voting problems is a theorem of Kenneth Arrow derived in 1951; see Körner (2008) for a thorough discussion of this transformative result. Pooling feature importances derived from several learning machines, as with merging voting preferences across many individual voters is, in general, doomed to generating cyclic conflicts of the form: a is better than b is better than c is better than a.

In a more classical statistical context, the ranking problem is also known to present nonresolvable conflicts. For example, we could be presented with a statistical procedure that ranks the merits of the output of three machines:

Machine A: 5.89, 5.98
Machine B: 5.81, 5.90
Machine C: 5.80, 5.99.

The data is taken from Haunsperger and Saari (1991). The *machines* here are not learning machines, but for our purposes they could be. Using the much-studied and broadly informative nonparametric Kruskal–Wallis (KW) statistical procedure, we rank the outcomes:

Machine A: 3, 5
Machine B: 2, 4
Machine C: 1, 6.

Under the KW procedure we now sum the ranks for the machines and find the ordering Machine A > Machine C > Machine B, as the votes are: A gets 8, B gets 6, and C gets 7. Now, we observe that an identical table of ranks is obtained under this set of output numbers:

Machine A: 5.69, 5.74
Machine B: 5.63, 5.71
Machine C: 5.61, 6.00.

But there is a problem when we attempt to pool the results into a single table of output values, where for example, Machine A will have the pooled values 5.89, 5.98, 5.69, 5.74. In the pooled table we find that the machines acquire the rank sums C: 30, A: 26, B: 22. That is, Machine A is ranked first under *both* of the two trials, but in the pooled data it drops to second!

The ranking problem then points to a deeper problem in the consistency of statistical inference. We don't offer any additional technical wisdom here, as there is provably no logical solution for the general problems just discussed. Getting *short* and more *interpretable* lists, with any ordering, is still an important practical goal, and learning machines are excellent for this more modest task. Finally, on a more hopeful note, if we change the terms of the merge problem slightly then progress is possible: see the intriguing work of Melnik *et al.* (2007).

Notes

(1) That is, a spine curved due to scoliosis may result in a tilting of the hips, causing one hip to rise and therefore the opposite leg to appear longer. Spinal curvature is in one sense a *static* clinical event, but it is closely related to, and better understood as part of the *dynamics* of walking. Let's dissect this problem as a way of understanding how features can work together.

One of the greatest assets of *Homo sapiens* is bipedal locomotion. The ability to stand and walk is a determinant of an individual's level of independence and health prognosis. It should not come as a surprise to learn that clinicians wish to monitor walking function, *WF*, for early signs of dysfunction. However, walking is a very complex task that requires the synchronized activation of numerous muscles in order to maintain balance against the pull of gravity and to control forward walking velocity. Like the spinal curvature example discussed previously, modern gait analysis techniques can be used to rigorously study a patient's walking characteristics, or *walking function*. Walking consists of identical cyclic patterns or strides of the right and left legs. Gait dynamics consist of the forces applied by the person walking, and to obtain the key walking measurements a pressure-sensitive device is built into the floor of a large room. Real-time motion-capture infrared photography can be used to monitor gait and position over time. The measurements then consist of left and right foot ground forces during walking, in two time points during each stride, for a total of four variables. It is found that the left leg force measurements, and separately the right leg forces, have correlations that are good predictors of normal walking function. There are also correlations between the left and right leg forces. Just as in the spinal curvature example above, all four features are essential for accurate prediction. Moreover, gait symmetry (or lack of it) is an alternative measure of smooth, normal walking. Hence there are at least two outcomes of interest and four interconnected features, and while strong correlations exist among the features, all are needed for good prediction.

Summarizing, this example highlights a series of independent clinical interpretations gained from a small set of closely related features. Study of the set reveals how the connections between the features have multiple clinical consequences. No single set of independently acting features can adequately predict the outcome. The features are coordinated, acting jointly, much as bipedal locomotion is itself.

(2) Epistatis is the occurrence of gene–gene interactions, is a wide-ranging phenomenon in biology, and indeed only a handful of genes (features) typically act in isolation. It also suggests that the idea of *function* in biology should have an expanded definition, certainly something far beyond simple additive or multiplicative functions; for more on this see, for example, Adami (2006) and Shao *et al.* (2008).

(3) This cardiac function model is mathematically similar to the one we just discussed for the pathologic spinal curvature problem. That is, for *CF* representing cardiac function, we can take the logarithms of both sides of the prediction equation:

$$\log(CF) = \log(A/B) = \log A - \log B, \tag{9.7}$$

and then define new variables:

$$LCF = \log(CF), \quad LA = \log(A), \quad LB = \log(B), \tag{9.8}$$

then the prediction model becomes linear:

$$LCF = LA - LB. \tag{9.9}$$

This has the same form as the spinal curvature model, where we let *SC* be the amount of spinal curvature measured for each patient, and *L*, *R* be the left and right leg lengths. Then:

$$SC = L - R. \tag{9.10}$$

(4) Partial correlation is mathematically well-framed, but not often used. Suppose, for example, we wish to see how variables 1 and 2 are related to each other, given that variable 3 is being "held constant." Given the correlations ρ_{12}, ρ_{13}, and ρ_{23} (or, estimates of them) the partial correlations are estimated using this equation:

$$\rho_{12.3} = \frac{\rho_{12} - \rho_{13}\rho_{23}}{\sqrt{\{(1-\rho_{13}^2)(1-\rho_{23}^2)\}}},$$

$$= \frac{0.80 - (-0.40)(-0.56)}{\sqrt{\{(1-(-0.40)^2)(1-(-0.56)^2)\}}} = 0.759. \tag{9.11}$$

Mathematically the definition derives from a correlation coefficient using the conditional distribution of the data, where outcomes for variables 1 and 2 are said to be *taken conditional on* variable 3. Such equations can be informative. The values of the partial correlations are closely related to the coefficients appearing in the usual regression equation, where we are interested in predicting variable 1 using 2, and 3. For details, see Muirhead (1982), Kendall and Stuart (1979, chapter 27).

We have seen the connection between features using correlations and found that simple correlations, such as ρ_{13}, ρ_{23} in themselves didn't capture the connections between variables 1 and 2 given by the simple correlation ρ_{12}. There is a special case when they can, namely when $\rho_{13} = 0$, or $\rho_{23} = 0$. Inspection of the defining equation above for $\rho_{12.3}$ reveals that in either of these cases, the partial correlation $\rho_{12.3}$ is then proportional to ρ_{12}, with $\rho_{12.3} = \text{constant} \times \rho_{12}$. Hence, if the simple correlation $\rho_{12} = 0$ then the partial correlation will be zero as well, $\rho_{12.3} = 0$. That is, the effect of holding temperature constant and evaluating the correlation between yield and rainfall is the same as that found when not considering the influence of temperature. We do not recommend depending on this more intricate correlation analysis as a method for sorting out connections between variables and outcomes, except in very small, known-to-be-linear models having just a few variables.

Moreover, there is a deeper question lurking for the scientist. That is, what does it mean (or, what should it mean) for a researcher to "hold" some set of variables fixed and allow another one (or sets of others) to vary freely. It makes sense in a factory, for example, where we can twist dials and machine settings at will and study the output of our Mark IV Widget assembly line. But this doesn't seem to make much sense when studying the effects of cholesterol, say, after "fixing" height, weight, and age for a patient: the patient who comes to the clinic can't be told to go away and come back when her height, weight, and age take on specific values. These values for the patient are random and specifically for height and age are not under her control. It could make sense to "fix" values if the model is intended to be used as part of an intervention, for which other measurements such as diet or level of exercise could be changed over time as part of a research protocol. Such interventions may be possible and sensible when, for example, a clinical trial is designed to study the consequences of increased exercise in two (otherwise identical) study populations. This distinction between pure observation and randomized, or interventional, studies is nontrivial.

The linkages between correlation, association, and intervention are complicated. David Freedman wrote extensively on this problem, its potential and more frequently, its hazards; see Freedman (1991, 1995, 1997, 1999).

(5) Here are two ways to understand R^2, the *coefficient of determination*. First suppose a model is given, such as Model 1 in the text. We don't worry for the moment about how the coefficients were estimated. Given the values for A, B, C, D, E, we can plug them in and calculate Y. Observe that this output value, call it $\hat{Y}$, is an estimate itself, since the model coefficients are estimated from the data. But the original data also has the observed value Y, linked to A, B, C, D, E. This yields a pair of numbers (Y, $\hat{Y}$) for each data point (Y, A, B, C, D, E). Collecting all these pairs together we can estimate a correlation in the usual way – then taking its square returns the number R^2; but see also Shieh (2001), Willett and Singer (1988).

Alternatively, the coefficient of determination represents the fraction of the total variance in the output y that can best be estimated from the data, using a linear regression model. See Draper and Smith (1998, chapter 1). Even with data that is well-fit using a linear model there are known cautions in using R^2. Here are two: by simply increasing the number of y-values observed at fixed values for the x-values (the predictors), the value of R^2 must decrease; and by simply adding more predictors, the value of R^2 again must increase even if the true coefficients in the model are all exactly zero; see Healy (1984), Draper (1984), Willett and Singer (1988).

Note that we're using this measure of accuracy for these linear regression models, and caution the reader strongly against using this particular measure for *nonlinear* models, in particular statistical learning machine models. Hence, even for a single classification tree, the coefficient of determination understood as either a correlation or a fraction of total variance, can be quite unreliable; see also Ratkowsky (1990, pp. 44–5).

Having given this warning it is also important to recognize that R^2 can be used rigorously, in some situations, when sufficient data is present. There is a well-developed literature on its use in validating logistic regression models. For more on this see Chapter 6, and Kuss (2002), Hu *et al.* (2006). It has been noted that R^2 is a statistical measure that statisticians love to hate, because of the toxic combination of widespread use and numerous essential, but unheeded cautions. Attempts have been made to rehabilitate it; see Anderson-Sprecher (1994).

An important detail about these equations: it is assumed that the features *A*, *B*, *C*, *D*, and *E* have been "centered" to have mean zero. This doesn't change our interpretive discussion here and makes for a cleaner-looking model. If this adjustment isn't made then the models shown in the text are equations that might be obtained under a "no-intercept" condition. This could be necessary and important for some experiments: we might want the consequences of very low contamination to be represented by increasingly low levels of harm, so that zero contamination means zero harm. In these cases the coefficient of determination does not have the simple interpretation just given.

(6) It is assumed that given the value of y, the xs are independent, Thus, for example:

$$\Pr(x_1 = 1, x_2 = 0 \mid y = 0) = \Pr(x_1 = 1 \mid y = 0) \times \Pr(x_2 = 0 \mid y = 0).$$

The conditional probabilities for this three-feature decision problem are given by:

$$
\begin{aligned}
\Pr(x_1 = 1 \mid y = 0) &= 0.1, & \Pr(x_1 = 1 \mid y = 1) &= 0.9 \\
\Pr(x_2 = 1 \mid y = 0) &= 0.05, & \Pr(x_1 = 1 \mid y = 1) &= 0.8 \\
\Pr(x_3 = 1 \mid y = 0) &= 0.01, & \Pr(x_3 = 1 \mid y = 1) &= 0.71 \\
\Pr(y = 1) &= 0.5.
\end{aligned}
\tag{9.12}
$$

With this starting information we find, after the usual, if tedious, calculations that values for the Bayes error are:

$$L(x_1) = 0.1, \quad L(x_2) = 0.125, \quad L(x_3) = 0.15,$$
$$L(x_1, x_2) = 0.0895, \quad L(x_1, x_3) = 0.069, \quad L(x_2, x_3) = 0.05875.$$

$$(9.13)$$

And these values lead to the inequalities quoted in the text.

(7) However, a practical distinction could be made in the cost per unit of observation in any of the models for any of the predictors. Is feature B harder to collect than feature A? Is measuring feature A consistently more accurate than measuring feature B? Does either of these considerations make Model 2 more practical than Model 1 or 3? Of course, in the case of A it presumably has the same cost per unit of observation in all three experiments, so the problem of sorting features according to costs per unit of observation or measurement efficiency, is difficult and often not resolvable. Such resolution requires embedding the original binary problem in a more fully elaborated *decision-theoretic* framework; see, for example, Hilden (2003, 2004).

(8) Our Figure 9.1 is a version of figure 3.20 in the comprehensive text of Seber and Wild (1989). Here are the two equations (models) for this data:

$$\text{Model 1}: f(x) = 7e^{-x/2} + 11e^{-x/7}$$
$$\text{Model 2}: f(x) = 11.78e^{-x/3.1} + 6.06e^{-x/9.4}.$$

$$(9.14)$$

Such similarities in these models (sums over exponentials) are well known among those who routinely deal with these models, and the problem in separating them is difficult. As a recurrent important problem it has a name, actually several, attached to it: this is the so-called problem of *identifiability*, and, its approximate version, *parameter redundancy*. Chapter 3 of Seber and Wild (1989) is an eye-opening journey through this subject.

(9) The superlative textbook on regression modeling by Harrell (2001, section 4.3) has a long, persuasive, and devastating discussion of this topic.

To more formally document some aspects of these problems, Freedman (1997, 1999) is a pivotal, beautifully argued study whose results have been replicated informally many times afterwards. The author began by generating outcomes from a set of 50 random variables, each of them having standard normal distributions and all uncorrelated with each other. The author then generated a 51st variable, also normal and also uncorrelated with all the previous variables. With this data so constructed, commonsense suggests that any sensible data-screening, variable-selecting method should come up with nothing of importance, since we have begun our analysis using data that is, to the best of our ability, completely content-free: simply noise. Instead, using a variety of feature-selection stepwise schemes, the author found that several small sets of the 50 (pure noise) features were selected, each with very high apparent predictive power. Applying the usual statistical tests, it was found that these subsets all showed highly significant R^2 values. It is one thing to rely on a procedure that sometimes misses important activity in the data, it is quite another to rely on one that routinely declares significance when there is, by design, no activity at all.

(10) This takes us to the large and broadly important subject of *model averaging*, and the use of decision rules that invoke some kind of ensemble or committee method. Such methods have been shown to be quite sound for many kinds of data analyses, and also have a Bayesian interpretation. See Chapter 12.

(11) There is a large literature on this subject, and it quickly takes the reader into some of the most important issues of the philosophy of science. It should be noted that in the history of science there are numerous important examples showing that facile applications of the razor can be seriously in error. Indeed, the atomic theory of matter proposed by John Dalton (1766–1844) and studied by Ludwig Boltzman (1844–1906) was rejected by Ernst Mach (1838–1916) and the logical positivists because it required adopting an entity – the atom – that was not seen at the time. The atom was, in this view, a complicating, unnecessary hypothesis: an uneconomical hypothesis. Continuing, proteins were once thought to be the transmitters of genetic information and DNA was considered for a time too complicating, as it required an apparently unlikely mechanical scheme for encoding and replicating. The idea here, as studied elsewhere in this book, is that what is "simple" is context-dependent and should be expected to change overnight.

(12) This is also a well-studied problem in social sciences, known as the voter preference problem; see, for example, Körner (2008, chapter 6). We will see Condorcet reappear in Chapter 12, when we study committee voting and ensemble methods. The important work of Saari (1995, 2008), Haunsperger (1992, 2003), Gintis (2009) should be noted. Important research in this area includes Fagin *et al.* (2003), Sabato and Shalev-Shwartz (2008), Ailon and Mohri (2008). For a promising line of research see Agarwal and Niyogi (2009).

Resampling methods

However beautiful the strategy, you should occasionally look at the results.

Winston Churchill

10.1 Introduction

In this chapter we discuss several basic computational tools, methods that have broad use in the data analysis community for a wide range of purposes. This is the class of sample reuse schemes, also known as resampling methods. These include *cross-validation* and the *leave-one-out* method.

Another key example in this class is the *bootstrap*, and in this text we use it extensively for obtaining improved estimates of prediction error rates. The method itself is very simple and easily explained. Why it often works so well is not so simple to explain but we make an effort, since improved comprehension in this area will help the reader apply the method in other data analysis contexts and sharpen awareness of its pitfalls.

We next consider much more computationally intense methods for improving on the apparent error rate, and for finding low-bias, low-variance estimates of almost anything.

Many of the ideas discussed here are ones that we've already needed to invoke in previous chapters, for example in discussing the Random Forests approach to error estimation, variable importance measures. So there is overlap here but this chapter provides additional detail, and is also a starting point for these ideas.

10.2 The bootstrap

The bootstrap method is an instance of *data resampling*. When applied to error analysis it is a generalization of the *cross-validation* and the *leave-one-out* schemes: these schemes are discussed here. For all these procedures we propose to reuse the available data after it has been collected but before we start to use it to make predictions on new data. We propose to reuse the data to effectively enlarge the apparent size of the dataset. It is possible to make this process very analytically rigorous and the virtues of resampling have been much studied in the statistical literature. As is typical for many intellectual innovations, resampling and bootstrapping was evidently used in the past, but only recently named as such from about 1979. Part of the research in this area has focused on identifying improvements to the methods, but equally importantly, it has identified instances when the methods don't do well. We consider both situations in this chapter.

We describe the bootstrap approach in stages: first we discuss how we can resample from the observed data, and then we discuss how repeated resampling can help us. Thus, first consider a set of five points (or other objects) labeled 1, 2, 3, 4, and 5. Suppose we sample from this set, pulling out one object at a time, and then replacing the object back in the set. This is called *sampling with replacement*. One such draw from the data could result in this set of integers: {1, 1, 2, 4, 5}.

We now discuss 10 aspects of this drawing scheme.

(1) Some of the labeled objects will not appear in our selection, and others might appear more than once.

(2) We will typically choose from the original set exactly as often as there are that many objects in the original set; five in this case. A shorthand description, therefore, of this process of generating the set {1, 1, 2, 4, 5} from the set {1, 2, 3, 4, 5} is this: we have done a single boot draw of size five. It is important to observe that doing boot draws of the same size as our original dataset is typical but not necessary. That is:

(3) In some circumstances we will make boot draws of size not equal to that of the original set. There are theoretical and practical reasons behind such choices and we considered these when discussing unbalanced data in Chapter 5.

(4) We make this boot-drawing process truly useful by doing it many, many times and, in one way or another, arrange to pool the results. Deciding to generate *six* boot draws of size *five*, we might have the following sets of selected objects:

$$B_1 = \{1, 1, 2, 2, 5\} \quad B_2 = \{2, 3, 4, 4, 5\} \quad B_3 = \{1, 3, 3, 3, 3\}$$
$$B_4 = \{1, 2, 2, 2, 5\} \quad B_5 = \{2, 3, 4, 5, 5\} \quad B_6 = \{1, 2, 3, 4, 5\}.$$

(5) Note that one or more boot draws may, in fact, reproduce the original data; in the sample just drawn, we find that B_6 is identical to our original data. This is not an error and no adjustment is required to the method.

(6) Since our draws from the original data are not weighted in any particular way (but could be in some circumstances), we can calculate explicitly the chance that any single point in the dataset is drawn in any single boot draw. The chance that any single point is selected in a single draw from a set of size n is therefore just $1/n$. If we make draws with replacement of size n from this dataset then the probability that a data point is *not* selected is about 36.8%; see Note 1.

(7) The data not drawn in a boot sample is not simply discarded in our analysis schemes, and indeed has a very practical, important purpose: it can act as a test or challenge dataset, and help improve our estimates of anything we've generated using the data that was in the boot sample. This use of the not-drawn data has a long history and has been shown to be very useful; see the discussion on Random Forests in Chapter 7.

(8) The data from which we draw the boot samples may be continuous (temperature, log gene expression, etc.) or discrete (SNP value, allele number, disease status, etc.). The bootstrap approach is applied to all such data in the same way: draw repeatedly from the given dataset, replacing points drawn after each selection.

(9) We have been considering samples that represent instances of a single feature or observation. The method of boot draws and resampling generally extends easily to data in which each instance is a vector or possibly long sequence, namely the values for each of many features. Data collected of this type may contain a long string of very diverse numbers and values, some continuous or discrete. When we do a boot draw from a collection of patient values we do so using the long string of values for that patient considered as a single data point in our draw.

It is important – but not necessarily obvious – that selecting entire strings of values, patient by patient, results in sets of strings that are boot draws over each of the values in the strings. Now, any correlation structure in the data is preserved when we do selections using entire strings at a time. This is an important aspect of boot drawing: we typically want to allow the individual features (values in the data strings) to collaborate, so to speak, in helping make predictions, classify or estimate.

(10) Despite the virtues of maintaining the internal structure of the data strings, it can be argued that it is better to break the correlation structure and let the features work separately as possibly weak but uncorrelated predictors. In fact, this approach underlies the frequently successful naïve Bayes machine; see Chapter 2.

10.3 When the bootstrap works

Having described the entirely mechanical process of generating subsets, we now describe the purpose of the method. Thus, it can be shown mathematically that, under quite broad conditions, generating such multiple subsets is something like generating new data, and so is something like increasing our sample size at very little experimental or computational cost. Here is why: when we resample from the data, using the sampling with replacement scheme, we are making selections from the data that automatically take into account the relative frequencies of the original data points. We are, therefore, sampling from a histogram, that is from an empirical distribution function. In the other direction, if we had an infinite supply of data, that is all possible data, then any samples drawn from this huge resource would automatically match the true proportions of all the possible outcomes. But since we don't typically have an infinite data resource – or can't easily simulate new data – we can make the assumption, provably valid or not, that our single sample from this infinite resource (Nature) is sufficiently representative, and then make a second assumption that resampling from the single observed sample is effectively equivalent to multiple samples drawn from Nature. The precise circumstances under which the multiple samples are approximately equivalent to multiple draws from Nature continues to be an object of mathematical study. Let's next consider an example for which the bootstrap method does not do well.

10.4 When the bootstrap doesn't work

A standard example for which the bootstrap does not work very well is the problem of determining the upper or lower boundary of a single feature in a dataset. Thus suppose we have data from the interval $[0, d]$, where d is an unknown constant, an upper limit for the data. We now draw a random sample of size 100 from, say, a uniform distribution of observations in this interval: every pair of small segments in the interval $[0, d]$ of the same length has the same chance of providing a data point in our sample.

This is our observed sample, and we proceed to do repeated boot draws from this sample. The important idea here: no amount of boot drawing will give us much information about the true but hidden value of d, except in one sense. That is, if the observed maximum in our original sample is 2.5, say, then we do know that the true value for d is at least that. But when the true value of d is 25.0 and the observed maximum is (still) only 2.5 – because our original sample remains fixed – then we won't detect anything close to 25.0. Nothing in *any* boot draw from this sample will help here.

We can express the problem slightly differently. Generating a confidence interval for an estimate of the upper limit of the data, using any boot draw data in our original sample is problematic: the upper end of the interval would essentially never cover the true value, d, unless that value was known to have some nonzero probability of occurring in any single sample (a weighted endpoint, in effect). So the basic problem here is that the bootstrap process can't be expected to be very good at estimating functions of the data that depend on extremes in the distribution. The bootstrap is also not very good (without some adjustment scheme) when asked to estimate particular segments of the data, such as the true upper 90% point in the original distribution, or the median of the unobserved population. This is the quantile estimation problem and the bootstrap research literature has a special section devoted to its solution; see Davison and Hinkley (1997).

We also know that the bootstrap is not very good, in its native unadjusted version, when asked to estimate some features of the data when the underlying distribution is not smooth and is, instead, clumpy (a mix of discrete and continuous outcomes, for example). Indeed, many technical proofs of the virtues of the bootstrap typically begin by assuming the underlying population is smooth (in the original mathematics, the underlying distribution function has derivatives of sufficiently high order).

Because of this potential problem the bootstrap has with not-smooth data, we find that a universe of alternatives has been offered, chief among which are functional data estimation and nonparametric density estimation schemes. In words, the first tries to estimate the entirety of some continuous, smooth function of the data, for example some centered, optimized path through the data; see Ramsay and Silverman (1997).

The second approach is quite classical and seeks to estimate the underlying distribution itself, rather than some aspect or property of the distribution. A modern treatment of this topic includes work by Biau and Devroye (2005), and the text by Devroye and Lugosi (2001). These are quite technical, but ultimately quite readable, being similar in spirit to DGL.

Both approaches are known to improve on the bootstrap in specific instances, but equally, both are analytically challenging, and they require input parameter choices by the user. They are, as well, often computationally difficult. The bootstrap, by comparison, is usually trivial to compute and generally requires few or no parametric choices. The exception to the lack of having to make parametric choices is the class of parametric bootstrap methods, wherein one uses good parametric estimate(s), of a mean and variance, say, and then boot draws are done from a user-specified distribution or model. If the model is well chosen, and the sample parametric estimates are good, then the parametric bootstrap can make a noticeable improvement over the so-called nonparametric bootstrap. However, in this text we will not use the parametric bootstrap, and the wise counsel of Davison and Hinkley (1997 p. 4) is very pertinent here:

Despite its scope and usefulness, [bootstrap] resampling must be carefully applied. Unless certain basic ideas are understood, it is all too easy to produce a solution to the wrong problem, or a bad solution to the right one. Bootstrap methods are intended to help avoid tedious calculations based on questionable assumptions, and this they do. But they cannot replace clear critical thought about the problem, appropriate design of the investigation and data analysis, and incisive presentation of conclusions.

10.5 Resampling from a single group in different ways

We have so far considered using the bootstrap for which the size of the boot draw, M, is equal to that of the original sample size, N. It might be asked, then, if this is necessary or efficient. That is, if many boot draws is useful why not just generate a single boot draw of size much larger than the original, say, a boot draw of $M = 500$ from a sample of size $N = 100$? This is an insufficiently examined research question, but there is at least one important situation in which we choose to generate boot draws of size distinct from the original sample size.

Thus, suppose given a sample of size N, we might be interested in choosing a new sample of size M, with M much bigger than N, sufficient to obtain high statistical power for a given inferential procedure. For this we could consider sampling with an increasing sequence of new Ms, $M_1, M_2, M_3, \ldots$, to study the improvements in statistical power; see Davison and Hinkley (1997, section 4.6).

Along this same line of thinking, we mention a simpler approach to dealing with the several problems of the bootstrap mentioned above, namely the failure of certain regularity conditions and study of data having heavy tails (extreme observations far from the center of the data). That is, interesting and pleasant consequences of doing a random draw, but not of same size as the sample, are presented in Ishwaran *et al.* (2009).

10.6 Resampling from groups with unequal sizes

Thus, so far we have considered just the basic mechanical problem of generating bootstrap samples for a single dataset. It is more often the case in biomedical research that we have data that is separated by various criteria, for example, a group of patients and another of controls. Such stratification of the data seemingly presents nothing new to the bootstrap, but a subtle problem can arise.

For the sake of illustration, consider the extreme example where the group of patients is of size 2 and the group of controls is of size 98, for a total of 100 cases under study. Suppose also that we wish to employ a method for making classifications of any new case into the disease group for which the patients are representative, or into the (normal) control group. Then the trivial method that assigns *every* new case to the control group, when applied to our dataset, will make an average error of just 2%. This seems impressive until we take it apart. That is, with this crude scheme we will be making an error of 100% on the patient group, and an error of 0% on the control group.

This is clearly unreasonable as a decision rule. If we want to use the bootstrap approach to generating datasets for training a decision rule, then we should expect to see this same kind of distortion in error rates if we don't account for the inequality of group sizes: we can't simply do boot draws from the total sample. Alternatives must be found.

This is the problem of unbalanced data, first mentioned in Section 4.5. There is now a considerable literature on the topic; see Wang and Japkowicz (2008), Jo and Japkowicz (2004), and the online bibliography dedicated entirely to the subject, Japkowicz (2009). A summary conclusion is that the better methods use a combination of several methods – over- and under-sampling – and systematic tuning by the researcher.

The problem intersects design issues that we take up later in Chapter 11. When we took apart the error estimate as above we were calculating the sensitivity and specificity of the decision rule. We were also ignoring questions relating to prevalence, that is how representative the two group sizes were in our target population: does the size of the at-risk group relative to the not-at-risk group accurately represent the importance of each in the general population? The comprehensive solution would take into account the typically competing error rates, sensitivity and specificity, and would also factor in estimates of the prevalence rates.

As mentioned earlier in this text, considerable effort has gone into sorting out the conceptual mix of user decisions about these rates and how to manage the associated costs of misclassifications; as just two examples of this subject, see for example Willan and Pinto (2005), Hilden (2003, 2004).

Example of unbalanced bootstrap sampling. We discuss the method of *undersampling.* We assume the costs of misclassification are equal for the two groups A, B, and that the incidence of the two groups in the larger population is equal. Suppose Group A is of size 20, and Group B is of size 100. Repeatedly draw bootstrap samples of size 20 from Group A, and size 20 as well from Group B. In the combined draw of size 40 we have a balanced sample, from which we can construct our decision rule. We will find that the group error rates will be approximately equal, and both equal to the overall error rate. On the other hand, we can anticipate that these error rates may not be especially good, since we are not using the data from Group *B* very efficiently: we're drawing at most only 20% from this group in each draw.

We note that the alternative approach, that of *oversampling* from the smaller group has been studied; see the literature on imbalanced data analysis given above. For this scheme, where Group *A* has *M* cases, and Group *B* has *K* cases, with $M \leq K$, we would generate a boot draw of size *K* from the smaller group, and a standard boot draw of size *K* from Group *B*. However, the research consensus appears to be that oversampling from the smaller group, in combination with the usual bootstrap sampling from the bigger group, is less efficient than the reverse, that of undersampling from the larger group and using standard bootstrap sampling from the smaller group. However, as noted above, combined methods, or over- and under-sampling seem to do best of all.

10.7 Resampling from small datasets

We don't always start with large datasets when we begin construction of a decision rule. Indeed, it is our experience in biomedical data that the cases of most interest, the patients say, form the smallest group: these cases are harder to collect, are infrequent in the general population, or both. Another frequent route ending in small sample sizes generally is that of microarray data. In this case we may have gene or protein expression outcomes for thousands, or even hundreds of thousands of genes or gene fragments or proteins, but have such expression data on just a few dozen cases. We expect the technology to soon provide us with millions of genetic and protein expression levels and SNP values, but not so soon to have hundreds or thousands of cases being sampled. The question then is the standard one: how do we best make use of the very limited or constrained data we do have? In our experience the bootstrap performs reasonably well if the data have anything to tell us in the first place. This is the standard answer to this recurrent statistical problem: if the underlying signal is reasonably strong, say if the patients and controls are easily separable under our decision rule, then our conclusions are robust and our error is low.

On the other hand, in Malley *et al.* (2003), we began with just 65 colon tumor instances from among 40 patients (with prone and supine scans for each), and a large collection of nontumor instances. Using a version of the bootstrap we sampled repeatedly from the 65 cases and found decent error rates, where the version used was one of a class of smoothed bootstrap procedures, the so-called 632+ method of Efron and Tibshirani (1997); see also Jiang and Simon (2007). To obtain good error rates, we therefore assist the process by smoothing the sample variance of the bootstrap error estimates. It has been noticed more generally that it is the observed variability of the bootstrap that suffers in small datasets, and this variability can be reduced with increased sampling and careful sampling design. When given a small dataset the bootstrap is still a viable scheme, but does tend to suffer from increased sample variance (basically as does nearly any statistical scheme).

The 632+ method is an interesting hybrid that owes something to the bootstrap technology and to the leave-one-out method discussed above. Technical results show that it (or still more refined versions) can meaningfully lower the sample variance of the estimated error rate, without greatly introducing bias into the estimate of the error itself; without inflating it or making it smaller and more optimistic. It has the additional virtue of being well suited to small datasets, for which some form of smoothing the error estimate is usually needed.

10.8 Permutation methods

An important family of methods that are similar in spirit to bootstrap methods, but predate it by many years, are permutation tests. Three texts in this area are Good (2005), Mielke and Berry (2001), and Edgington (1995).

Here is a simple experiment outlining the method. Following Good (2005), suppose we have concluded an experiment on cell cultures, generating six growth plates from a single cell line. On three of these plates we had added to the standard growth media, a compound that contains vitamin E, thought to extend life (at least by those still living to vouch for its wondrous properties). On the three other we plated the cells using only the standard growth media. We wait a number of days, hoping that no plates become inadvertently infected with other growths that might affect our chosen cell line. At the end of the waiting we are relieved to see that all six plates have survived intact, and we count the cell concentrations on all six plates.

We find the following cell concentrations, in suitable units:

121, 118, 110, 34, 12, 22.

Primed now to see the obvious benefits of vitamin E, we recall the identity of the three plates with the additive and the three without.

Biologically we say that if we had not added vitamin E to any plates, or equivalently, if the result of adding vitamin E has no real effect on cell growth or longevity, then all six plates should seem rather similar at the end of the waiting period. Otherwise expressed, if we divide the six plates into two groups of three each, we should find that an arbitrary division this way should result in cell growth numbers similar to those found if we had measured the three with-E plates against the three without-E plates.

Given the assumption of biological equivalence across the six plates we now choose a computational benchmark for gauging cell growth across a set of plates. As Good (2005), and others very accurately point out, there should always be some time and thinking devoted to choosing this figure of merit, since we are always having to include both statistical efficiency and scientific relevance in the choice.

In this case we decide to take the total cell growth (as measured using a radiological tag) across each set of three plates. The set of three plates for which we did apply the vitamin E treatment had a cell total of 349: {121, 118, 110}.

We proceed to randomly divide our six plates into all possible groups of three. For example, {121, 118, 34} and {110, 12, 22}. The sum over the first set is 273, and the sum over the second is 144. Note that the total across all six always remains fixed at 417, so we need only keep totals for one of the groups.

We continue randomly dividing the six plates into sets of three and counting the total cell concentrations in each group. There are exactly 20 such divisions into two sets of three, and the 20 cell counts for the two groups, starting with the highest, include these:

first group {121, 118, 110} and second group {34, 22, 12}; first group total = 349;
first group {121, 118, 34} and second group {110, 22, 12}; first group total = 273;
... and 18 other arrangements with smaller totals, the smallest being 68.

Here is the next interesting step in this permutation approach: *if* vitamin E truly has no effect on cell growth or longevity, and *if* otherwise the cell counts are statistically equivalent then the cell total we got on our first arrangement, 349, should be completely unremarkable in our complete list of possible 20 cell totals. That is, in the observed listing of all possible cell totals, we would expect that the value 349 would not appear as unusually low or high, and would appear as such only rarely. The reader can probably now see the parallel here with familiar statistical testing methods: under a null hypothesis of no difference (however that might be biologically defined), we expect to find the observed outcome (statistic based on the data) to show up in the lower or upper tails of the distribution with a probability calculated from the true distribution. In our case we have only the complete listing of outcomes (the full listing of 20 cell totals).

With our original cell count, 349, in the extreme upper tail, it is in the top $1/20 = 0.05$ of the cell count listing. Borrowing from the frequentist approach to statistical hypothesis testing, we can conduct a one-tailed test of our null model and declare that 349, being exceeded by no other observations, is a rare event. More precisely, the structure of this kind of permutation testing suggests we declare our observed 349 as evidence that the null model should be rejected at the 0.05 level.

Note that we might be on firmer ground if we note that any significant departure from the null model would drive our observed count to the extreme upper *or* the extreme lower end. Under this interpretation, we would assume a null model with a two-sided symmetric hypothesis, where we see if our observed count occupied either the upper tail or the lower one. Therefore, we would declare our cell count significant at the $0.05 + 0.05 = 0.10$ level.

As usual with formal statistical testing, the practitioner is required to be quite specific and careful about what is being tested and what could be expected under the non-null, or, alternative models. Our decision about the benefits of vitamin E for these specific cell lines is a function of certain choices, each of which are open to meaningful disagreement. In the discussion of Good (2005, p. 9) the case is made for testing the model under a one-tailed hypothesis, and he declares the vitamin E growth factor to be significant at the 0.05 level. He also goes on to confess that the apparently significant results from this one experiment were never obtained again in his several replications of the experiment. Perhaps a two-tailed test should have been applied? But this discussion should not obscure an important aspect of this permutation method, namely that we have not had to specify further any other statistical part of the testing scheme. In particular, we have not had to make any parametric, or distributional assumptions.

The somewhat less appealing feature of this procedure is that we have to be rather careful in how we state the results we obtain, specifically, we cannot assert that our outcomes immediately generalize to the hypothetical (mythical?) population of all cell growth plates. We are, after all, only studying the behavior of a single sample, so we need to be careful in stating that the result obtained is representative in any important way of the larger hypothetical sample of all possible six-plate, vitamin E growth experiments. It is a matter of some technical controversy as to whether, or how easily, this generalization is valid or even relevant, but ultimately the central biological argument has to be that the experiment needs to be replicated, using new cell plates, more cell growing and counting.

Let's assume that the permutation approach has some capacity for useful generalization, for a given experiment. We can, for that experiment, then proceed to test any number of useful statistical aspects of the data. We consider two such applications.

10.9 Still more on permutation methods

To apply the permutation procedure for testing group differences we can follow a general outline given in Mielke and Berry (2001), this time applied to multivariate data. As with the cell growth, vitamin E experiment, we start by assuming the null model, of no differences in the groups. Scientifically we assume that the long list of features attached to each subject (cell plate, for instance) are samples from some (possibly very high-dimensional) distribution, whose shape and other features are not known to us. Therefore the only difference across the cases are the group labels, which under the null model are entirely arbitrary: there really is only one group.

To conduct the expanded permutation procedure we invoke one of the methods called Multiple Response Permutation Procedures (MRPP), as defined in Mielke and Berry (2001). Therefore, the next step is to select some measure of distance between any two of the cases. This is a novel aspect of the

MRPP approach and is rather different from the selection of a single group statistic, such as the sum over the cell counts in each of the two sets of three plates. The MRPP approach argues that if the groups are distinct, then the typical or average case-to-case *distances* in the groups should be smaller than the case-to-case distances across any random pair of cases in the entire dataset. Note that case-to-case distances within a group are closely related, but crucially different from the within-group measure used in analysis of variance, namely the sum of squared differences for each case, from the within group mean. The squared differences used in conventional analysis of variance are known to be sensitive to unusual cases, those that are unusually far from the within-group mean. Also, it is possible to argue that the actual Euclidean distance $d(i, j)$ is a more accessible measure for the researcher than the squared distance between cases i and j, which is equal to $[d(i, j)]^2$. To be sure, there is a substantial literature on choosing the distance measure for each problem, and the outcome of the permutation test hinges on this choice to some degree.

We have now completed the most important intellectual aspect of this expanded permutation procedure, the choice of case-to-case distance measure. We then proceed to run the procedure just as we did with the cell-grown vitamin E experiment, by randomly switching all the labels, but still keeping the group sizes the same, and calculating the distance measure for each permutation of the dataset. A list of the permuted measures then yields an observed histogram of outcomes, and we locate our original distance measure in this plot. If the original distance calculation is in the top 5% of the list of outcomes, say, we argue that if the groups are truly distinct (in the distance measure we chose), then a statistically rare event has occurred, *or*, the groups must have been distinct in the first place.

Several comments need to be made at this point.

First, it is common for the many measurements that have been made on each of the cases, the features for the problem, not to be made in the same scale. We could have, for example, x_1 measured in centimeters, x_2 measured in microliters, x_3 measured in decibels, etc. Any single summary measurement of the distance between cases will reflect this lack of equality in scale and commensurability. If the sample variance for x_1 is 100 times that of the sample variance for x_2, then the distance between cases will be greatly affected by small differences in x_1 and much less so for differences in x_2. This is a standard problem for any single summary score across heterogeneous features. Mielke and Berry (2001) suggest using transformed versions of the features.

Second, we have recommended above that a permutation test of the global hypothesis of any difference in the two groups be performed using the complete list of features. Now, similar to the problem of features with greatly differing scales and ranges, is the problem that the groups might be provably different but only so in some small fraction of the complete list of features. The small set of group differences in this case would find itself buried in the big set of noisy, nonseparating features. How to locate just the useful differences?

This question takes us back to a problem we considered much earlier, in Chapter 7 – that of determining the importance of the many features under study. So it seems we haven't advanced the game very far. But let's note that a plausible feature selection method can be used first, and then the permutation test can be applied to the smaller, more refined feature list. Thus, the problem of uncovering group differences using a very long list of features, is entirely tied up with the problem of determining those few features that, jointly, most effectively distinguish the groups. We do not offer a singular solution to this problem – it is an essential problem of experimental science. We do encourage flexibility in any approach, and all plausible approaches should be *mutually reinforcing*, for the concluding inference to be considered successful.

Third, we haven't discussed how we might weight the cases for the (standard) situation in which the group sizes are unequal. Mielke and Berry (2001) discuss this in some detail and find that, for the two-group case (such as we generally consider here), the group weights and the ultimate weighted distance measure, for group sizes n_1, n_2, should be calculated using:

$$C_1 = \frac{n_1 - 1}{K - 2}, C_2 = \frac{n_2 - 1}{K - 2},$$

$$\xi_1 = \frac{2}{n_1(n_1 - 1)}, \xi_2 = \frac{2}{n_2(n_2 - 1)},$$

so that the final distance value is:

$$\delta = \xi_1 C_1 + \xi_2 C_2.$$

Fourth, it will usually be the case that the complete list of all possible permuted cases is enormous and any calculation of case-to-case distances across all the permutations would take much too long. As a practical alternative we typically only generate some small subset of the total list. This subset can still be very large, but usually the calculations are fast, so we can routinely generate a million permutations. The point here is that this is a form of Monte Carlo testing, and can fairly quickly approximate the true permutation test value.

Here is how we can apply permutation methods in the statistical learning machine context, for making predictions about two groups, at-risk and not-at-risk, say.

We calculate the error rate for the original data with the correct group labels. We permute the group labels (as in the vitamin E experiment) and apply the same prediction engine to the two groups, and record the error for this permuted data. If the engine is truly better than coin tossing, we would expect to find, as in the cell growth problem, that the error rate we obtained on the dataset with all labels intact should be a rare event. Note here that we truly have a one-sided testing environment, as the null model is that the error rate should be that of coin tossing, namely an "accuracy" of 0.50. If our learning machine is working well, our original error rate should be appreciably distant from 0.50. For a sample of three cases in Group A and three more in Group B, we find just as above that there are 20 possible divisions of the data randomly into Group A and Group B. If our observed rate is the lowest among the 20 instances in the permutation distribution, then, just as before, we can declare our prediction engine better than coin-tossing, at a $1/20 = 0.05$ level.

Note that this method works even if the apparent error rate, using the correct group labels, is not very auspicious, say 0.30. In this case we may or may not be able to separate the outcome using the correct group labels, from the permuted data. If we do find that the 0.30 rate is rare among all the permuted outcomes, then we can claim that the machine is probably not doing random coin-tossing when it makes predictions. But the biomedical value of a procedure with a 0.30 error is probably not very great. In our experience we don't highly promote a machine that makes a validated, carefully confirmed error of 0.30 or more.

Moreover, as with any form of statistical testing or estimation, and in particular permutation testing, we need to think very carefully about what is, in fact, under test. Loosely speaking, the method just described has a composite null hypothesis: it is possible that our prediction engine is actually quite good, but that for the dataset we use to study it, is simply not very informative. In this case no engine can be expected to strictly outperform random coin-tossing. The parallel here with the cell-growth problem is that the statistic we *chose* to evaluate cell growth, the sum over the three plates, may not be the appropriate, most sensitive method for the scientific problem. Or, it might be the best method for general cell growth problems but is being applied to data in an experiment, and those particular cell-growing conditions, that isn't especially sensitive for measuring cell growth. Or, again, the vitamin E additive might be biologically irrelevant for cell growth, or for the particular cells we chose to use. This can all be very difficult to sort out. An obsessively complete listing of possible interpretative problems is our suggested strategy in this situation, as well as a listing of possible positive conclusions under the assumption that the results are valid.

Finally, we need to be careful in how we arrived at the particular prediction engine we want to study using this permutation approach. It is best if we generate the engine using data that we then do not use for the permutation testing. Otherwise we run the risk of using the data twice and falling prey to the problem of overfitting. One scheme for dealing with this is to first generate a boot draw from the two groups, *A* and *B*, generate the prediction engine on the boot draw, and then test it on the data not in the boot draw (the OOB data). The Random Forests, and Random Jungles, learning machines both include this method as standard. If not already part of the learning machine of choice in your lab, it should be.

Note

(1) In large datasets, the probability that a single item (object, subject, data point) will not be selected is the limit $(1 - 1/n)^n \rightarrow 1/e \approx 0.368$. Here, e is the mathematical constant $2.71828 \ldots$ (and many more digits, besides). In words, the portion of the data *not* selected in a boot draw (of the same size as the original data) is approximately 36.8%, which means that the proportion of the data that *is* selected in a boot draw is about $(1 - 0.368) \times 100 = 63.2\%$.

Error analysis and model validation

The aim of science is not to open the door to infinite wisdom, but to set a limit on infinite error.

Bertolt Brecht[1]

11.1 Introduction

In this chapter we show how the performance of a single learning machine can be evaluated, and how pairs of machines can be compared. Our focus will be on evaluating the prediction error of a machine, that is, how often it places a subject in the incorrect group, case or control, say. We immediately state that the problem of estimating the accuracy of a machine designed for predicting a continuous outcome (temperature, say) is a different and ultimately harder question. A very brief discussion of error analysis for continuous outcomes is given at the end of the chapter, but as stated in Chapter 2, we don't spend nearly enough time on this important problem.

After covering prediction error for a single machine we then examine how any pair of machines can be evaluated: is one significantly better than the other? This kind of paired analysis applies to the comparison of one familiar statistical engine, say logistic regression, with a nonparametric, nonlinear prediction engine such as Random Forests. In this case the comparison is between a big, somewhat hard-to-understand machine and a little, relatively well-understood one. Our analysis of single machines and sets of machines will introduce three ideas.

First, for evaluating a single machine it is good and standard that an estimate of the prediction error should be accompanied by a confidence

---

[1] ©Bertolt Brecht, *The Life of Galileo*, Methuen Drama, an imprint of A&C Black Publishers Ltd.

interval, or some other variance-related estimate of the reported error estimate. Simply reporting a mean value for the estimated error, even after doing possibly thousands of runs in a simulation, is simply not enough. However, using simulations to globally validate any machine, with the aim of justifying its use over any other machine, is usually mistaken, unless the assigned task for the machine is to predict data for which the researcher has precise and detailed knowledge of its statistical (distributional) properties; see the discussion on *benchmarking* in Sections 2.11 and 11.13

Second, also important is the study of the large-sample behavior of the error estimate. That is, does the method used for estimating the error behave well as more data is collected. An error estimate that is always strongly optimistic (low apparent error relative to true error), or, that is wildly varying from one sample to another, is not well behaved in this sense. We point out that an optimistic error estimation scheme need not lead to an incorrect selection of a machine from among a set of possible prediction engines: it might instead mean that the error estimation method is not well adapted to the machine under study. We discuss this below. An error estimation scheme with high variability is a different problem, however, and selecting from among a small collection of machines is undermined in this case.

The more mathematical sector of the machine learning community has worked on these intertwined ideas, of bias and variance, for decades. We can therefore report on some of the more conclusive or intriguing of these findings. The point here is that this deep technical literature offers guidance on what to expect of any error estimation scheme for learning machines.

Third, for comparing two machines it is essential that the evaluation take note of the usually nonremovable correlation built into the comparison. That is, a good comparison of a pair of machines requires asking them to make a prediction on each case, or subject, and this necessarily generates *correlated* outcomes. Taking account of this correlation is straightforward, once it is recognized, and indeed we can quote from the recent statistical literature on paired comparisons to implement methods that are markedly better than widely used classical ones.

11.2 Errors? What errors?

Suppose we apply a learning machine to a single dataset. We want to evaluate its predictive performance and this requires, at a minimum, getting a low-bias, low-variance estimate of its true error. Additionally, a confidence interval for the true error is informative and should be standard.

We introduced basic definitions in Chapter 4. For a given subject a machine makes a prediction (classification) and it's either correct or incorrect. The *observed error* estimate is given by the number of incorrect predictions divided by the number of subjects with which it was presented. This simple error estimate can itself be quite in error if it was derived using the same data as was used to generate the machine under test. This result is a version of the overfitting problem; more on this below.

Additionally we need these two measures, sensitivity and specificity, which are coupled in the following sense: we could identify every truly at-risk subject by declaring all subjects to be at risk, but then we would also be incorrectly naming many healthy subjects as at risk. Similarly, if we identify no subjects as at risk then we never make the mistake of misclassifying a healthy subject, but then we're never catching any at-risk subject. Either approach is extreme and problematic, unless the costs of misclassification have been sifted carefully into the analysis.

All these statistical measures can be expressed in terms of the four entries of the so-called confusion matrix; see Table 11.1.

The sensitivity, specificity, error rate, and precision are expressed in terms of these four numbers, T_P, T_N, F_P, F_N:

$$\text{sensitivity} = \frac{T_P}{T_P + F_N}$$

$$\text{specificity} = \frac{T_N}{T_N + F_P}$$

$$\text{overall error} = \frac{F_N + F_P}{T_N + T_P + F_N + F_P} = (F_N + F_P)/n$$

$$\text{precision} = 1 - \text{overall error} = \frac{T_N + T_P}{T_N + T_P + F_N + F_P} = (T_N + T_P)/n.$$

Table 11.1 Calculating sensitivity and specificity

	Sick	Healthy
Classified sick	True positive = T_P	False positive = F_P (Type I error)
Classified healthy	False negative = F_N (Type II error)	True negative = T_N

11.3 Unbalanced data, unbalanced errors

In many datasets, the number of subjects in the two outcome groups is not the same: there are more patients who survived than did not, and more survivors who regained functional independence than survivors who did not. These are examples of unbalanced datasets, and are quite common in biomedical research: the number of positives (not at risk, controls, etc.) is often far larger than the number of negatives (at risk, cases, etc.). This is often true because the at-risk cases are harder to collect, are more clinically rare. Such is the case with the lupus data, with only 109 negatives out of 3839 subjects. We first covered this topic in Sections 4.5 and 10.6.

Suppose we ignore the inequality of the group sizes and simply trust the learning machines to reveal any predictive power in the data. We will often find that several machines obtain remarkably low error values, as was shown in Table 4.2, with errors about 3% for all of the machines except LDA, which had errors of 23% and 40% when the BIGSET and RFIMP predictor sets were used.

Examination of the sensitivity and specificity for these machines, all having low *overall* error rates, shows that the sensitivity of each of the methods is extremely low, while the specificity is close to 100%. The learning machines are evidently teaching us that it is always "safer" to declare a person healthy, since the proportion of not-healthy people in this data is very low: $109/3839 \approx 2.8\%$.

This is a mistaken approach, of course, and we do not need this kind of help, from a human expert or a machine. We want both high specificity and high sensitivity. Any single one of these measures is not enough to responsibly quantify the performance of any learning machine.

In fact, unbalanced data presents a difficulty not only for learning machines in general but more specifically for any OOB or bootstrap or resampling method. Briefly, the problem is this: when we do a sampling with replacement from unbalanced data, the probability that we sample from the larger group is naturally higher than for the smaller group. But then if we test on the data that remains – as we do in OOB – the larger group will still be much larger compared to the smaller group, so we're back to the unbalanced data problem we just described. That is, drawing a sample of size 50 from a group of 1000 leaves behind 950 for OOB testing, and drawing 50 from a group of 100 leaves 50 behind for testing. Most machines, or human deciders for that matter, will now prefer to err on the side of caution and declare in favor of the larger group exactly as we saw above, when only the overall error rate is being evaluated.

In using OOB and resampling methods we need to monitor both the proportion of sampling from very unequal groups (for machine training) and the proportion of data left behind (for machine testing). However, while there does not seem to be a universally approved method for balancing data prior to error analysis, we suggest two methods.

(1) *Ratio sampling*, where the ratio between the positives and negatives is fixed to be the same in the original dataset and the bootstrapped dataset. This could be used when the observed ratio is assumed to match the population incidence of the two groups. Including population incidence information is a more sophisticated technique and in this analytic realm we probably should also include information on the cost of misclassification.

(2) *Total balancing*, where the number of negative and positive cases used for learning and testing is forced to be equal. One way to do this is by undersampling (also called downsampling) from the larger group, thus generating a sample for testing that is approximately equal to the size of the smaller group.

11.4 Error analysis for a single machine

As a routine matter of sound statistical practice it is essential that once a decision rule has been generated, we need to spend nontrivial amounts of time and brainpower determining if the procedure is usefully predictive and deriving some assurance that the estimation of the errors is itself robust.

For background on this subject we find that an excellent, very detailed discussion of learning machine error estimation is given in DGL (chapters

22, 23, and 24). Here are three other excellent texts covering the error estimation problem, specifically directed at classical biomedical data analysis: Zhou *et al.* (2002), Hand (1997), and Pepe (2003). We strongly encourage looking into these comprehensive works – there is much sound error analysis to be found therein, that we are omitting in this book.

To see some of the problems involved in getting good error estimates, let's start with the basic *observed* (or *apparent*, or *resubstitution*) error estimate mentioned above. It has long been noted that simply calculating the observed error value for the very same data that was used to generate the decision rule leads to a biased estimate, one that doesn't have on average the true error value for that rule. It often happens that the apparent error estimate is exactly zero, and too often this can be seen as the value appearing in published reports. This is a silly estimate, of course, but the deeper statistical problem here is specifically that the bias of the apparent error estimate is nearly always positive – the decision rule looks too good, with an estimated error that is too small. DGL (chapter 23) has a detailed probabilistic analysis of the optimism driving the apparent error value.

That this quick and natural estimate is sharply optimistic partly explains its still widespread use. But as noted above, consistently optimistic bias is not necessarily an evil property: comparing *two* machines using such an estimate can still lead to correct selection among the pair of machines, since we can see that the difference in their error values could be maintained given any bias, up or down.

Here is a dramatic example – given in DGL (p. 398) – that makes clear the optimism of the observed error. Suppose we decide on using a *k-nearest neighbor* decision rule and in fact use $k = 1$; see Chapter 3 for more on these rules. Now, for this machine, when given a test data point the rule operates by locating the nearest neighbor of the test point in the data already collected, and then declaring the group membership for the test point to be assigned that is the known group membership for this neighbor. Then estimating the observed error for this rule, we are to take as test point each of the original data points, one after the other. But, the single nearest neighbor to the test point is – the point itself! And as its distance to itself is exactly zero, certainly no other point can be closer. Hence the group decision for the "test" point is exactly the group identification of the point itself, and the group memberships for these "two" points are always in agreement. But then the apparent error is zero for all the "test" points. This error estimate, for this machine, is returning zero information.

Several comments are in order. These comments are translations from theory and practice, and are dark, cautionary tales for the most part. Once we step outside the tidy world of small models with data models having well-understood parametric form, the analytic universe becomes quite fluid and surprising. On the other hand, see Note 1.

First, the problem with the observed error estimate in this case cannot be laid at the door of an inefficient parameter estimation process for the classifier – *any* k-nearest neighbor rule has exactly zero parameters that strictly require estimation before being applied to a dataset. And very simple versions of these rules – the one-nearest neighbor scheme – can be shown to do quite well. This is another example of primitive but excellent. Of course, the researcher might want to optimize this choice in some way using the data, so that the prediction error is low, or becomes low as enough data is collected.

Second, getting an estimate of the typical error for a given machine is usually dependent on the often-complex coupling between the machine and the data itself. Some machines might have better error estimation using one method rather than another. The point here is that an absurd estimate of the error made by a machine (as in the one-nearest neighbor scheme) is not the same as asserting that the machine itself is not predictive for a given distribution.

Third, while the one-nearest neighbor error estimation example is striking and worrisome, the mathematical fact remains that the observed error estimate can still be shown to be very good with only some slight modifications; see DGL (chapter 23).

Fourth, recall from Section 2.11 that for any machine there are prediction problems (datasets) that require astronomical amounts of data to yield predictions with low error. This is true even when, by construction, the machine is known to achieve the optimal Bayes lower limit for prediction for a distribution. And this negative finding holds even in the situation where the true minimum error is exactly zero (that is, the groups are fully separated; see DGL (chapter 7)). This result must compel our attention, and we restate it: suppose we are given any small positive number, say 0.05, any machine, and any given sample size N. Then there always exists a dataset (distribution) such that the true error made by that machine on that dataset, for that sample size, is within 0.05 of the coin-tossing rate of ½. And this distribution is, indeed, such that by construction the true Bayes error is exactly zero.

Fifth, it is possible that two machines, both with low error values, can have *identical* error rates and yet make distinct predictions for individual subjects. For this, imagine a very simple problem (distribution) where there is a sharp boundary separating two groups, cases and controls. And suppose that the two machines have slightly different estimates of the boundary, such that a few cases or controls are misassigned by one machine, and the other machine misassigns a different set of cases and controls. If the numbers of misassignments are equal for a dataset then the observed errors will be the same overall for both machines. And it might be possible that the cases being misassigned are not equivalent in terms of clinical or biomedical consequences; we need to think about this with every new dataset.

With these translations and warnings in place, we turn to the practical problem of getting good error estimates, starting with the family of cross-validation methods. These reuse the original data but in ways that can be shown to be relatively unbiased, so that overfitting is reduced. The general topic of *sample reuse* was discussed in Chapter 10.

11.5 Cross-validation error estimation

Consider a dataset with 20 subjects, with 10 cases and 10 controls. Assume we have a machine learning scheme that has been generated on this dataset of 20 subjects. We are interested in getting good estimates of the true error for the scheme, and only have the 20 subjects available for this analysis. One simple method is as follows; see Note 2.

The two-fold cross-validation (2XCV) method. Randomly divide the 10 cases and then the 10 controls into two equal groups, A and B, say, each of size 10, each containing 5 cases and 5 controls. Apply the method for generating the learning scheme on Group A, obtaining Scheme A, say, and then apply the method to the Group B cases. If on this test dataset we make b mistakes, this yields an error rate of the form ($b/10$). Next, apply the method for generating the scheme to Group B and then test on Group A, obtaining a mistakes, and an error estimate of $(a / 10)$. In all, this yields $[(a + b)/20]$ as an overall error rate. Then we conclude with two actions: we report the averaged error value for the learning machine, and declare the machine being used under test as that generated by applying it to the original 20 subjects.

The 2XCV method is still widely applied in the biomedical literature, but in fact probably should never be used. It has one serious drawback, that of large sample variance compared with other methods. Indeed, the sample variance of the error estimate can often be large even when the actual error estimate is on average fairly close to the true error value. For example, a sample mean taken over just two data points has a large sample variance compared to one taken over 10 data points, even though the average over a very large number of such two-data-point estimates would be nearly unbiased: that *average* coud be close to the true error value. Ideally we want the error estimate to be on average close to the true value, and we also want the sample variance to be small. That is, it is required to have a relatively unbiased estimate and some interval that contains the true value with high probability.

One natural alternative to the two-fold cross-validation is this: the mXCV method, where m is much larger than 2. Often an m of just 5 or 10 yields low variance and relatively low bias. The numerical scheme for the 5XCV approach is parallel to that for the 2XCV. Begin by randomly dividing the data into five segments, train on the first four segments, and test (get an error estimate) on the remaining fifth segment. Repeat this, each time training on a different segment of four, and testing on the segment left out.

For any of the mXCV methods just outlined we issue the following caution. It is critical that the m segments (for $m = 5$ or 10, etc.) be truly random segments of the complete set of subjects. We could expect unusual or odd results if, for example, we inadvertently placed all the high-cholesterol cases in just one of five segments in an application of the 5XCV method. One way to ensure such randomization is to let our computer make a segmentation of the data, but even then it is still useful to look over the segments so generated for anomalous specialization: the high cholesterols aren't ending up in mostly just one segment.

And this randomization issue just discussed now suggests a more systematic alternative: instead of cleanly dividing the data into m distinct segments, choose a training dataset having a fixed proportion of the data, say 90%, and do so repeatedly. Here we would randomly choose 90% of the total subjects, generate a decision rule on that 90% sample, test that rule on the 10% omitted, and then continue choosing, randomly, new subsets containing 90% of the cases. We would report the average error over all these many test sets, and report the machine scheme obtained using the complete data.

Several comments are pertinent at this point . . .

11.6 Cross-validation or cross-training?

As the reader may already have detected in the above discussion, we have intermingled the process of *estimating* the error of a machine with the process of *generating* the machine itself. This is problematic, for several reasons, and the issues here are complex, but not insuperable.

First, the error analysis just described is the reported estimate of the true error for the machine generated using all the data, and it is not the elementary estimate of the error for that machine as applied to all the data (that would be the observed error). The reported error based on cross-validation is derived from versions of the machine as generated using smaller segments of the data. As such, the machine versions are being constructed using less of the data, so are themselves probably not as accurate as a machine generated using all the data. Nonetheless, results from theory show that cross-validation is a sound procedure for machine error analysis.

Second, closely related to the cross-validation method for error estimation, it is possible to consider using the data to help select from among a family of (possibly very different) learning machines, using part of the data set aside for (so-called) *training*, and then using the other part of the data for *testing* the machine, or, estimating the error for the selected "best" machine. Technical details and large sample bounds on the error estimates are presented in DGL (chapter 22).

Third, this process of using training and test data is quite widely applicable and is not limited in theory or practice to getting estimates of the error: training and testing can be a foundation for generating a machine. Indeed, there is a substantial technical literature on how a classifier can be optimally selected from among a family of classifiers. This testing and training approach is called *empirical risk minimization*. Casually dropping a term like this in many social situations will impress, confuse, or simply irritate; use with caution. And the most deeply considered, general version of this approach is *structural risk minimization*; see Chapter 3, DGL (chapter 18), and Vapnik (2000).

Fourth, there is a subtle problem lurking in the shadows here, one that is indeed a little hard to describe even free of mathematical gears and levers. Namely, if we use all the data in some resampling scheme to generate multiple versions of a machine, and then test each on left-out data, or on some testing dataset, then we aren't exactly evaluating a single machine, but generating multiple error estimates for multiple machines. Each of these generated machines will be slightly different, and lead to slightly different predictions for the same subjects, since they each see different portions of the data. Hence there is some resampling variation in the "single" machine under test. In fact, under this scheme there isn't any single machine under test, but many. The question then becomes: do we want to evaluate a single machine, for application to the next subject appearing in the clinic, or should we focus instead on how all those features appearing in the multiple machines are being utilized. Does the next subject care what the entire class of all possible machines of some given type does with her clinical values?

We don't presume to have a single answer to this last problem; it remains as another Canonical Question. But it has been suggested that this variation – generation of the machine itself – must be included in the process by which we evaluate the "final" machine; see Varma and Simon (2006). Under this approach, of resampling and repeated generation of a machine, and then repeated testing on the left-out data, the bias (optimism) and variability of the prediction error is evidently reduced, for at least some well-parameterized distributions and datasets.

Leaving aside the precise details and numerous variations, there are three basic steps to this process of empirical risk minimization, the use of training and testing data.

(1) A collection of classifiers is chosen by the researcher, and this family can be quite large indeed. It can include many different kinds of prediction

engines (many types of nearest neighbor, trees or many species, parametric models of all sorts).

(2) The data is divided into two parts, with one portion called the *training data* and the remaining part the *test data*. The training data is used to select a single machine from the collection, using some form of empirical error estimation.

(3) The remaining, test data is used to estimate the error for the selected classifier.

We note that the training data can also be used to estimate any parameters or other required values for any single machine, while the test data is typically used to generate the simple observed error estimate. As the training data is assumed to be statistically independent of the test data, there isn't any serious problem with optimism in the observed error estimate as we saw above.

We next consider other, often computationally intense, methods for improving on the apparent error value, methods that are more likely to yield low-bias, low-variance estimates.

11.7 The leave-one-out method

A simpler, but more time-consuming alternative to the *m*XCV method is this: select one case of the dataset, use all the remaining data to train the machine, and then test the machine on the single case. Follow this up by working through the entire dataset, leaving one case out, training on the remaining cases, and then testing on that left-out case. Under this method each case gets left out and tested exactly once. There isn't any problem over which segments of the data are being used for training and then for testing: checking for true random selection is not a problem. It is known that this method (called the *deleted error* estimate in DGL) usually has low bias: on average it will accurately estimate the true error. However, it has a somewhat high sample variance: repeated samples of the same size will generate error estimates with relatively large variation. There have been numerous improvements suggested in the literature for this method that appear to retain the low bias and drive down the variance. These approaches are usually (computer) labor-intensive, but do work well in practice; see Note 3.

11.8 The out-of-bag method

Here is another computer-intensive approach to error estimation. We introduced it first in Chapter 4, where we analyzed three datasets. And the bootstrap method for estimation generally was discussed in Chapter 10, being an instance of data resampling. This method is similar in that respect to the mXCV and the leave-one-out methods, just discussed. Implementation of the bootstrap works this way: do repeated boot draws from the data, generate a machine, and apply it to the data not selected in the boot draw. Breiman introduced a version of this idea in the Random Forests machine, naming it OOB estimation.

Note that with this method:

(1) the machine is not being tested on totally distinct segments of the data (as the data is used repeatedly in each boot draw), and
(2) a given subject may reappear in more than one boot draw and also in more than one OOB segment of the data.

Despite the fact that the training and testing segments are not distinct, the OOB approach is considered quite good; schematically it straddles the two methods we've discussed above, cross-validation and leave-one-out.

On the other hand, any bootstrap method is in a sense rather wasteful of the data, simply because the probability of never selecting some points (and then leaving them out-of-bag) is itself not equal to zero: in every boot draw about a third of the data will not be selected. Do we really want to generate a machine using only about two-thirds of the data, and then test it on only the other one-third? The simple answer from *experience* is no, probably not. Yet the bootstrap approach within OOB doesn't use just two-thirds and one-third this way, and instead uses hundreds (or thousands) of fractions of the data. As shown by theory, it is this extreme repetition and overwhelming resampling that drives the bootstrap approach toward efficient (low-bias, low-variance) error estimation.

Finally, a very important point about the OOB scheme and bootstrap estimation generally, one that is perhaps not obvious: for very unequal numbers of cases and controls the method can lead to very biased estimates of sensitivity and specificity – see the discussion below on unbalanced data analysis.

Table 11.2 Out-of-bag (OOB) and Monte Carlo (MC) error estimates for several machines on the simulated cholesterol data. Each analysis uses 100 runs of newly simulated data, or 100 OOB computations

Machine	Error rate % ± one standard error	Sensitivity % ± one standard error	Specificity % ± one standard error
Simulated data			
Neural net with 50 hidden units	0.81 ± 0.42	96 ± 2	100.0
k-nearest neighbor with $k = 5$	1.6 ± 0.58	93 ± 3.2	100.0
Boosting with 100 iterations	2.5 ± 0.59	89 ± 3.1	99 ± 0.4
SVM radial basis	2.1 ± 0.65	89 ± 3.7	100.0
CART	3.4 ± 0.84	86 ± 3.7	99 ± 0.54
Linear discriminant	34.0 ± 2.2	82 ± 4.2	63 ± 2.4
OOB using original data			
Neural net with 50 hidden units	0.95 ± 2.2	97 ± 2.7	99 ± 3.5
k-nearest neighbor with $k = 5$	2.7 ± 1.2	92 ± 6.2	99 ± 0.9
Boosting with 100 iterations	3.5 ± 1.5	89 ± 7.7	98 ± 1.5
SVM radial basis	3.7 ± 1.5	82 ± 8.2	99 ± 1.1
CART	4.7 ± 1.8	85 ± 9.1	97 ± 1.4
Linear discriminant	34.0 ± 3.7	75 ± 7.2	64 ± 4.7

In Table 11.2 we present results for error estimation on the cholesterol data, using both the OOB and the MC method. As seen, while the linear discriminant scheme has relatively large error values, the OOB and simulated data estimates of these values are quite close.

11.9 Intervals for error estimates for a single machine

We should routinely use large numbers of OOB runs, getting an average and a standard error. The estimated standard error even for a good prediction engine is an essential property of reporting on performance. The next important step in evaluating any learning machine is deriving an interval for the estimate. We would like the interval to behave, in large samples, as does a familiar confidence interval: with some stated probability, the true value of the error used for that machine is contained within the displayed interval. In the absence of parametric models for the machine itself, a large sample interval having a specific probability of containing the true error is problematic; see DGL (chapter 30) for more technical details of error analysis for machines. However, not having a precise, assumption-driven interval is not the same as having no pretty good interval. Approximate methods are always available and serve nearly the same purpose as classical confidence intervals. There are three settings for generating these intervals.

First, if sufficient data is available, the machine can be generated (selected, estimated) on the training data and then evaluated on the test data. Under the standard assumption that the data points are statistically independent, the test data will provide a sample mean and variance for the observed error. The sample size of the test data is then used in the standard way to generate a confidence interval for the true mean of a (binomial) random variable.

We suggest a minimum of 30 data points in the test data for generating this classical interval. This choice of 30 is drawn entirely from our data experience; it doesn't stand up under mathematical examination. A more careful, sharper analysis always depends on the signal strength in the data, and this is itself generally unknown. The strength of the signal in the data and the choice of method used to detect it can require far fewer data points, or thousands more.

Second, if fewer than 30 data points are available for training and testing, interval generation is more problematic. Thus, the leave-one-out (deleted) estimate can be used along with the sample size of the dataset in a classical binomial interval, but the predictions made for each of the n data points are not statistically independent: the n machines are generated on overlapping portions of the data, and are themselves not independent. A similar criticism can be made for any form of cross-validation. In place of the classical interval for a binomial random variable we can use the observed error for the deleted estimate and a sample variance calculated *as if* the predictions were independent.

Third, for the OOB approach or the bootstrap method generally, it is good to compute the observed average of the estimated errors (made on each of the many out-of-bag samples), and calculate the standard error of these estimates. There is a separate literature on how the bootstrap can be used for confidence intervals and for error analysis; see Davison and Hinkley (1997, chapter 5).

Fourth, and finally, much more evolved estimates are possible and have been studied extensively for any of these approaches based on using the data for both training and testing. In general, some form of smoothing of the many error estimates is suggested, along with corrections that attempt to reduce the apparent optimism of these estimates; see Note 4. It is also true that extended, highly evolved refinements on error analysis face diminishing returns: if the signal is strong in the data then the error value (and its associated standard error) will be small using almost any method of estimation, and if it isn't then the error value will look more like random coin-tossing (error value approaching 0.5), and no refinement will make the picture any prettier.

On the other hand, notice that we have focused on error values under a weak but lurking assumption that the data does have *some* signal in it, that is, the true error value is respectably far from coin-tossing. If the error value is above about 0.30, say, then another path needs to be taken. That is, we need to check if the machine is really doing no better than coin-tossing. . .

11.10 Tossing random coins into the abyss

If the estimated error for a machine is high, say above 0.30, then the apparent signal in the data is weak. But now the question is: just how weak? Is the machine just doing random coin-tossing, for which we expect to be right about half the time, or is there some really slight signal in the data?

Here is one scheme for estimating our proximity to the abyss:

Step One.   Generate a machine and record the associated error value using the original data.

Step Two.   Randomly relabel the original data – randomly rename a case as a control, and a control as a case.

Step Three.   Apply the original machine to the relabeled data and record the error value (using the original error method as in *Step One*).

Step Four.   Do *Steps Two* and *Three* many, many times, each time recording the observed error value; call this number of times n.

Step Five.   Bookkeeping: count the number of times, m, the relabeled analyses are equal to, or less than, the original error value; calculate $c = m / n$.

The value c is the proportion of instances in which the permuted data reveals more signal (using that specific machine) than the original, unpermuted data. It is a Monte Carlo permutation estimate of the significance of the signal in the data, under the null hypothesis that the original data is, itself, random (that is, contains no signal at all, for which the true error value, C, would be $C = 0.50$).

If additional data is available, separate from the training data, then this test data can be used for the permutation testing as above. If the observed error value is below 0.30 then it may be less necessary to do this evaluation, but it is never inappropriate to do so. Estimating proximity to the abyss is good statistical practice.

We point out that checking for the appearance of random coin-tossing can be a productive step independently of error estimation. Suppose, for example, that a microarray project has generated SNP data but it seems possible that there is a plate, or batch effect. In this case, if the normal controls appear all on one series of plates and the cases on another series, then a learning machine applied to the two groups might declare only weak predictions. It could be argued, however, that the plates themselves were too variable and inconsistent, and any data signal was masked by a batch effect.

To check this (that is, to use learning machines to evaluate *data integrity*), we can apply the coin-tossing method itself, more or less exactly as above. Thus, any two plates that are known to both contain only cases, or only controls, should *not* be separable using any good machine. Having generated a machine on the original data (two plates of cases, or two plates of controls), and noted the estimated error value, we proceed to permute the labels on the two plates, as in the *Steps* above. In this case, we would expect to find that the original error value is surrounded by all the permuted error values, and basically only very infrequently would any permuted value appear lower than the observed value. Again, this is a simple Monte Carlo permutation test of the null model, but in this situation we would expect to find that the null model is not rejected: the two control (case) plates are not separable.

11.11 Error estimates for unbalanced data

In using any of the methods described above for estimating the error of a machine there is a natural hazard, often of considerable practical consequence. This is the problem of unbalanced data, for which the group sizes (cases, and controls, say) are very unequal. A study of not balancing data for a range of machines as applied to the lupus data was given in Table 4.2. These results are, and should be, disturbing.

In general, we would rather have nearly balanced sensitivity and specificity. This equal weighting of the two kinds of errors will change as we probe deeper into the costs of misclassification and the true proportions of cases and (normal) controls in our target population. Such cost/benefit analyses and reasoning from prior probabilities (for group membership) are undeniably important in biomedical decision-making; see Pepe (2003). And see also (section 32.3 of DGL).

As mentioned at the beginning of this chapter, there is a hidden hazard present in unbalanced data when any of the bootstrap-based methods are used for error estimation. The problem is this: if we start with 90 controls and 10 cases, we can consider doing a boot draw of size 90 from the controls and size 10 from the cases to generate a machine. If we use the OOB method for error estimation we then use the cases not selected in either draw to estimate the error of the machine. Here we are using (on average) 6 of the cases and 60 or so of the controls for the test: the testing sample sizes derive from the fact that a bootstrap on average has approximately a 62.3% chance of drawing any given subject. But now the very unequal test samples will once more lead to error estimates that greatly favor the larger group, in this instance, the 60 controls over the 6 cases. Then, repeated boot draws in the OOB process will *not* correct for the lack of balance, and only reinforce the bias.

There is another version of this problem with unbalanced data analysis and error estimation. For some machine-learning schemes, the data is reused repeatedly to generate the machine itself by making repeated estimates of the incurred error and suitable adjustments to the path of the machine generation. This happens, for instance, in the Random Forests approach and indeed in some widely used versions of the basic single tree scheme as well, where features are selected for incorporation into the machine (tree or trees) on the basis of a rapid on-the-fly estimate of the predictive usefulness of each feature compared with others. For these forest and tree methods the error estimation is being done using the OOB scheme, which we have seen above is not so good when the data are unbalanced. Any learning machine that tightly hooks together machine generation (estimation of parameters, tree node splits) with feature selection based on error analysis will have to confront this problem.

A simple expedient for the OOB scheme and similar bootstrap procedures is just to send only balanced data to the program that generates the learning machine of interest. This usually means some elementary preprocessing of the data: generate multiple (possibly thousands) of balanced datasets containing equal numbers of cases and controls, and send these datasets to the program that generates and tests the learning machine of interest. Collecting the many estimates of the error using these multiple versions of the data will provide an approximate average error for sensitivity, specificity, and sample standard deviations for both. This bookkeeping requires careful programming scripts and coding, but seems to work well in practice.

11.12 Confidence intervals for comparing error values

A critical part of evaluating any machine is its comparison to some other machine, or, classical statistical decision-making scheme. We would like, for example, to detect signal with a learning machine and then move to a smaller, better-understood procedure (one with far fewer features, for example) and still track the drift in error. For this we borrow from classical statistical methods the notion that when two sets of observations (random variables, estimates) are paired, then an efficient method of comparison should take into account the correlation of the observations; see Note 5.

Some basic data analysis comments help motivate this approach. If the observations have positive correlation then a comparison of the two mean values of the observations could be based on the *difference* in the observations, with an adjustment made for the correlation. Alternatives such as ratios of the error values, or an odds ratio in a matched-pairs analysis, could be used as well.

For comparing any pair of statistical learning schemes, we can expect that a pair of methods will generate positively correlated outcomes when applied to each subject. Most importantly, two learning machines that are both pretty good will typically be making the same prediction on each subject, namely the *correct* group classification, and hence will tend to be positively correlated. And perfectly accurate machines (both with zero error) will have perfect correlation in predictions, so that as error values are driven downward we need to account increasingly for the correlation.

Having established the importance of paired comparisons that take advantage of positive correlation, we are happy to report that recently many new statistical methods have been developed that improve sharply on the construction of confidence intervals for the difference in error values. Starting with Tango (1998), a flood of new methods have been introduced that correct for such problems with classical methods. For example, an interval that includes values outside the range $[-1, +1]$ is not possible in theory for any difference of the form

$$\{\text{estimated error for machine } A - \text{estimated error for machine } B\},$$

whenever the estimates are both in the interval $[0, 1]$. And just as important, the new methods have also been shown to more accurately contain the true difference in the error values. Tables 11.3–11.5 display a worked example of a pair of such methods (Wald and Tango) using the Stroke-A data for training two machines and the Stroke-B data for testing and applying these methods. See Note 6.

Since the two 95% confidence intervals in Table 11.6 do not contain the origin – but nearly do – we see that using just the top 10 features in a

Table 11.3 The confusion matrices for Random Forests as applied to Stroke A, using all 38 features, and then using the top 10 features. Outcome 0 = full restitution; outcome 1 = partial or no restitution

All 38 features		0	1	Top 10 features		0	1
	0	488	192		0	462	218
	1	153	527		1	156	524

Overall error: (153+192)/1360 = 0.2537   (156+218)/1360 = 0.275

Table 11.4 Matched-pairs table for two Random Forests machines, one using all 38 features on Stroke A, the other using the top 10 features

		RF using all 38	
		0	1
RF using top 10	0	542	99
	1	76	643

Table 11.5 95% confidence intervals for the difference in error rates using RF (all 38) and RF (top 10), obtained from the adjusted Wald method and the Tango score method

Adjusted Wald:	[−0.017497, −0.016277]
Tango score:	[−0.017521, −0.016303]

Random Forests analysis is not quite the same as using all 38 features. We might have suspected just this conclusion from the error analysis in Table 11.3, where the top 10 error rate is 0.275, while that for all 38 is 0.2537. Whether this detected difference in the two machines is biomedically significant is another story, and one we don't take up here.

Applying the adjusted Wald or the Tango methods is simple enough (using the R code) but, as with any error analysis, it is important to keep in mind two things; how the data is used, and if the data is unbalanced. Thus, a simple leave-one-out approach could be taken, where a pair of machines is (repeatedly) generated on all but one of the subjects, and then applied to the left-out subject data. Or, a cross-validation scheme could be used. The proviso here is that each machine makes a prediction on each subject exactly once. That is, an OOB error estimation approach would not obviously satisfy the statistical requirements of the Tango (or other) method for getting a confidence interval for the difference in error values: the paired predictions for the machines would not be statistically independent if all the subjects reappear in the list of predictions.

Our concerns expressed above about getting single error estimates for *unbalanced* data carry forward into any discussion of confidence intervals for the difference in error values for any pair of machines. If the data has been separated into training and testing segments then the Tango (or other) procedure for machine pair evaluation can be applied directly with the testing data. Alternatively, we suggest simply sending the prediction machine-generating code only for multiple, balanced datasets, and then summarizing the multiple error estimates as means with a sample variance. See Note 7.

11.13 Other measures of machine accuracy

There is a very large statistical literature on evaluating prediction schemes, where a prediction is derived from a variable threshold approach. For example, a single logistic regression can be used to make binary predictions by choosing a cut-off in the estimated log odds (given by the model) for each subject. This was first discussed in Chapter 5. Indeed, any machine that leads to binary predictions by choosing a cut-off (as in voting schemes) can be studied using the technology we now discuss: *receiver operating curves* (ROC) analysis.

This process is simple enough: for each cut-off a specific binary prediction engine is being defined, and hence can be evaluated in terms of the two kinds of errors that are possible – sensitivity and specificity – the errors made in prediction for each of the two groups. We can plot sensitivity along one axis and (1 – specificity) along the other axis, for some large range of cut-offs.

Here is the important technical insight: shortly after ROC analysis was introduced, it was observed that the area under the ROC curve was related directly to a nonparametric test statistic for the difference between the two groups being classified, when the difference is measured using the range of cut-offs selected in generating the curve. This is admittedly convoluted as a statistical procedure, but does make a certain sense. If the area under the curve is close to one (its maximum possible value), then the prediction engine is doing very well at every cut-off of interest: it is making only small errors in classifying either group, using the full range of cut-offs.

And then more generally, a statistical comparison of two machines can be made using the difference in the areas under the ROC curve for each machine.

ROC methods are widely used, but do have some important problems; see Note 10. We discuss two of these:

(1) The area under the ROC curve – its AUC – is a global summary of how a machine does using all possible cut-offs. For example, we could study an ensemble or committee machine evaluated using all possible voting thresholds across the collection of machines, from m votes out of a possible n votes, where m ranges from $n / 2$, say, to n. Otherwise expressed, the area under the curve approach is an evaluation of an *entire family* of prediction machines, with each family member determined by a cut-off value.

However, in practice, in making a diagnostic prediction for the next patient coming into the clinic, or the next possible tumor cell type in the lab, we probably are most interested in using a *single* machine, one for example that has equally small misclassification errors of each kind (false positive and false negative). That is, we need to select a cut-off and choose that single machine for prediction. In this light, global summaries such as an area are not of much help: a procedure could be quite acceptable for one cut-off and not so good for another, and in practice we're only interested in making a single optimal selection of the cut-off. Another version of this fact is that the ROC curve could be quite unacceptable in regions of the plot of (sensitivity, 1 – specificity) but we won't be operating (making predictions) under those parts of the plot.

(2) Using the area under the ROC curve has another problem: it can be shown to be (effectively) a Wilcoxon rank sum test of the difference in location of the two groups, when each subject of the group is scored

using the value of the machine at the selected cut-off. Note that in the case where every subject is given some value of a continuous number, such as in logistic regression and log odds for each subject, then the Wilcoxon rank sum value is the sum of the ranks assigned to all members of one group, where the ranking is done on the combined group data using the continuous outcome. See, for example, Sprent and Smeeton (2001).

If it is known that the collected predictions for the two groups, when scored this way, are indeed different in *only a location shift and in no other way*, then this familiar rank sum test is sensible and often more powerful than the usual *t*-test. However, simple examples show how it evolves into something not sensible if, say, there is a difference in within-group variances along with a shift in location. While the Wilcoxon rank sum test does not require the two groups to have a given shape in any sense (such as a normal bell-shaped distribution), it does assume that the only distinction in the groups is a pure change in location. It is possible to evaluate the accuracy of this location-only assumption, but the inference then gets highly conditional upon the outcomes of the screening tests. In our experience a typical ROC analysis rarely encourages this basic evaluation, either exactly or approximately.

Given (1) and (2) as above we currently don't recommend using ROC analysis for evaluating any single machine, or choosing between any pair of machines. This is admittedly a somewhat minority view, and for more on this see Milden (2003, 2004). More broadly, consult Bossuyt *et al.* (2006), Guyatt *et al.* (1992), Monton and Guyatt (2008). A penetrating technical analysis of ROC also occurs in the discussion of *proper scoring roles*, for which see Gneiting and Raftery (2007).

11.14 Benchmarking and winning the lottery

It is very common and entirely natural that given a single machine we would like to demonstrate convincingly that our chosen approach is just that good and globally thus. So, often, we proceed to collect other data and compare results using other machines. This is a deeply flawed approach, and any statements of the true moral excellence for one machine over another derived this way are necessarily suspect.

Here is the simple reason, which we recall from Section 2.11. From theory it is known that for any given learning Machine A there always exists a distribution, and another Machine B such that the error probability of Machine B is lower than that for Machine A. Indeed, we can find Machine B such that it is, for these data, Bayes consistent for that distribution, in fact universally consistent; see DGL (p. 5). Winning the machine lottery is always data-dependent, and we can't win the machine lottery every day of the week; there are provably no super-classifiers. Multiple machines need to be applied and collected and assessed, and on each dataset (distribution) the winner is just that, the *data-specific* winner.

This result, from theory, answers Canonical Question 20, as given in Chapter 1.

However, this gloomy assessment is distinct from another conclusion very close by, which is not very gloomy at all. That is, studying how a pair of machines behaves on a single dataset, or on multiple datasets, can tell us how those machines actually perform and can be understood. The worked examples in Chapter 4 have this goal in mind: reporting on the inner workings of several machines, but avoiding the trap of declaring a universal winner. Looking ahead to Chapter 12, we will find that combining machines avoids the problem of having to declare any single machine as a winner.

11.15 Error analysis for predicting continuous outcomes

We have not spent much time in this book dealing with machines that make predictions for continuous outcomes, apart from the important special case of machines designed to predict the probability of group membership. This probability in principle could be *any* number in the interval [0, 1], so such a probability machine naturally qualifies as one that outputs a continuous prediction. The more general one of predicting something like temperature or the measurement of total cholesterol is the topic of regression analysis. We direct the reader to other texts for this topic, such as the excellent Harrell (2001), and the more technical Györfi *et al.* (2010).

Two comments are in order.

First, one of the standard methods for evaluating a regression machine (one making continuous predictions) is its (estimated) *mean squared error*, MSE. Most basic statistical texts discuss the definition of MSE and its interpretation. However, essentially all the discussions are being made in the setting of a known probability specification for the features and the outcomes in the data, such as the multivariate standard normal distribution. The standard properties of the MSE, or the usual adjustments to it, can become completely unwound and unverifiable when we take even a slight step away from this much-studied, tidy universe. The estimated MSE can, for one example, become negative: what do we make of an error estimate that is less than zero? Chapter 9 discussed the closely related value, R^2, as one way to approach this problem.

Second, many pure regression engines can be turned into classification engines by segmenting the output of the machine into, say, high and low measured outcomes. In this way we exchange the continuous outcome for a group identification, and then can apply any of the methods described above to the problem. Quite reasonably, we would expect any sensible regression engine to also do well as a (transformed) prediction engine, with low errors under each form of the machine. While we don't undertake the next interesting question (of how to jointly link the two kinds of errors), lack of agreement between the two measures should be a cautionary finding. As a practical matter when given a continuous quantity to predict, we can apply several segmenting methods to the output and confirm that the errors and results are similar to what we find using the original continuous form of the outcome.

Notes

(1) It can be shown that *if* a good rule (a Bayes consistent rule) happens to be in the collection of machines under consideration, then the *train + test scheme* will also then deliver a good rule (DGL, theorem 22.1, p. 289).

(2) Cross-validation is also called the *rotation method*; see DGL (p. 556). Results from theory and practice show it to have somewhat higher bias than the leave-one-out method, described in the text above, but also showing smaller variance.

(3) The leave-one-out method can be shown to be universally quite good given enough data. One of the most important results from theory is undoubtedly this: suppose we chose to apply a k-nearest neighbor rule $g(x)$ and we're given a dataset of size n. Let the true (but unknown) error for the rule on a given dataset be denoted $g(x)$ on a given dataset be denoted L_n. And suppose we choose to use the leave-one-out (deletion) method, L_n^D for estimating L_n. Then on average, over all samples of size n from this distribution:

$$E[(L_n^D - L_n)^2] \leq \frac{6k+1}{n} .$$

For details, see Rogers and Wagner (1978), Devroye and Wagner (1976). In particular, consider this error bound for the primitive *one*-nearest neighbor rule, which like any nearest neighbor rule, doesn't involve any "training" or parameter estimation or adjustment at all: it has an expected mean squared error relative to the true error for the method, that is at most $7 / n$.

Another version of this kind of upper bound for nearest neighbor rules is this. Let L^* denote the Bayes error value. That is, the best possible error value for any possible machine. Next let L_{NN} denote the error made in very large samples with the nearest neighbor rule. Then simply and remarkably:

$$L^* \leq L_{NN} \leq 2L^*.$$

That is, *if* the Bayes optimal error for *any* conceivable learning machine, on any dataset, is small, say equal to 0.05, then given enough data the *one*-nearest neighbor rule will be in error at most 10%. Numerous improvements have been made to this bound originally devised by Cover and Hart (1967), and understood as well by a subsequent extension due to Stone (1977); see also DGL (chapter 5). We comment that this series of theoretical results was responsible historically for a significant movement toward the current understanding of how learning machines can and cannot perform well.

(4) Given our focus on error estimation in this chapter, we return to a statement made earlier in Chapter 2 on linear discriminant methods. Two comments are in order.

First, the separation between two groups has a specific definition in the setting of linear discriminants, namely the Mahalanobis distance, for which see DGL (p. 30). This is a weighted measure of the distance of any test point to the means of the two groups, where the weights account for the overall shape (covariance) of the data. Suppose now we adopt the conventional assumption that each of the two groups has multivariate normally distributed data. It then follows that a larger (weighted) distance between the means of the two groups implies a sharper separation of the groups, and thus a better chance that the linear discriminant method will have a lower overall error of misclassification. However, in general this does *not* mean that the true Bayes error for the problem is smaller. Thus, a quite general (theoretical) upper bound for the linear discriminant error shows that it does go down as the distance increases, but this error could still be far from the Bayes lower limiting error value; see DGL (p. 57). It is interesting to note, however, that this quite general upper bound for the linear discriminant classifier is exactly twice that for the large-sample nearest neighbor rule. A provocative but still reasonable question to ask is this: is it *ever* plausible to use a fully parametric linear discriminant as a learning machine instead of something as simple as a nearest neighbor rule? One reasonable answer, that sidesteps the original question, is that an ensemble approach that combines a linear discriminant machine with a handful of others, including a nearest neighbor machine, is a safer approach: see our discussion on committee methods in Chapter 12.

Second, it is possible to construct datasets of arbitrary size such that the linear discriminant rule has error arbitrarily close to one, but for which there exist *other* linear classifying rules that have error arbitrarily close to zero. Indeed, for such data, a linear support vector machine (as described in Chapter 2) will have this essentially zero error value.

(5) The efficiency of taking differences when making paired comparisons for positively correlated outcomes derives from this standard bit of statistical theory. The variance of a difference is given by:

$$\mathrm{var}(A - B) = \mathrm{var}(A) + \mathrm{var}(B) - 2\mathrm{cov}(A, B),$$

where $\mathrm{cov}(A, B)$ is the covariance for the pair A, B. In case A and B are positively correlated this term is itself positive, and in turn this means that

$$\mathrm{var}(A - B) \le \mathrm{var}(A) + \mathrm{var}(B).$$

Hence a procedure derived from the difference between A and B will be more precise on average than based on A and B used separately. This is an example of blocking as used in the statistical theory of experimental design.

(6) The abundance of newer methods for making paired comparisons apparently began with Tango (1998). This and related issues were then later ably surveyed by Newcombe in a long series of important papers (1998a,b,c, 2006a,b, 2007). Much progress continues to be made in this area, once considered complete and "settled" by the original Clopper–Pearson method dating from 1934; see, for example, Zhou and Qin (2003). Here we are applying an adjusted Wald confidence interval and the Tango score interval, using the R code as described in Agresti and Min (2005).

(7) There is an interesting research problem here: given that we have available many confidence intervals for the difference in error values for a pair of machines, is it possible to generate a single, summarizing interval or region? Such multiple intervals could be generated, for example, from a great many boot draws of the data, with each draw yielding a Tango interval. Each interval is described as a pair of endpoints containing at least approximately some high probability of surrounding the true difference in error values. We *conjecture* that the following scheme will have good, large-sample statistical properties: as a single 95% confidence region, find all those points that are contained in at least 95% of all the confidence intervals. This will be computationally intensive and is not certain to yield a single, unbroken interval. However, we can expect to find that all but a finite number of intervals will be bounded from above by some point, and this scheme will then give an estimate of maximum difference in the error values of the two machines.

(8) We gratefully acknowledge that our understanding of this topic was enormously expanded by numerous discussions with Professors. Jørgen Hilden (University of Copenhagen) and Paul Glasziou (University of Oxford).

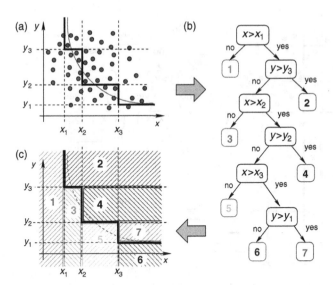

Figure 6.5   One way to slice up the data.

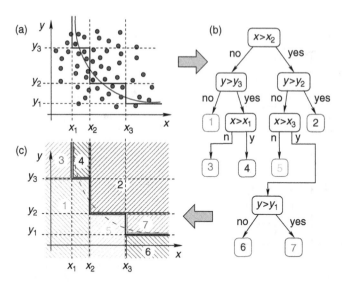

Figure 6.6   Another way to slice up the data; or is it?

Part IV

Machine strategies

12

Ensemble methods – let's take a vote

How full of inconsistencies, contradictions and absurdities it is. I declare that taking the average of many minds that have recently come before me, I should prefer the obedience, affections and instinct of a dog before it.

Michael Faraday

12.1 Pools of machines

The wisdom of groups has been much studied. The jury system for legal decision-making is one practical example of this notion. However, why can a group be wise, or more precisely, when can a group act wisely and when might it not, is the real issue for us. Thus, theoretical studies lead to so-called ensemble methods, or committee decision rules, as often provably better than single classifiers. This research reveals not only the wisdom of group decisions, under certain carefully noted circumstances, but much more: groups can act quite wisely even when individuals in the group are not especially wise at all. That basic classifiers which are not particularly good when acting alone, can when acting jointly become quite good, is not at all intuitive. But this insight leads to an important class of decision-making tools, and we discuss the wisdom of ensembles in this chapter.

12.2 Weak correlation with outcome can be good enough

In Chapter 8 we introduced the idea that predictors that are only weakly correlated with the outcome can, acting jointly, be quite strong. This certainly seems counter-intuitive, but has been known for some time, since at least 1785; see Note 1. Indeed, this relative lack of correlation (with outcome) across even very weak decision-makers leads to an important design endpoint for constructing a learning machine. This idea is invoked explicitly in the Random Forests approach to statistical learning; see Chapter 7. Let's study this in more detail – it is a foundational idea.

Consider a collection of 19 decision-makers, which we formally characterize as 19 binary {0, 1} features, $\{A_1, A_2, \ldots, A_{19}\}$ such that each is a predictor *by itself* of some binary outcome variable B. (The curious number 19 is chosen to avoid the problem of split decisions; any odd number would work for our argument, but even numbers work as well if we invoke some split decision rule.) So, while we have 19 possible predictions when presented with the data, *how* each prediction is made using the *same* data is unknown to us for the moment: indeed, it's not even relevant for our argument. Let's next assume that using any single feature by itself results in the high prediction error of 0.30, for example. That is, 30% of the cases will be misclassified in using any single feature A_i and each feature in itself is a pretty weak prediction engine.

Assume next the predictors are essentially statistically independent, or at least they are uncorrelated among themselves, $\text{cor}(A_i, A_j) = 0$. We now form a prediction scheme on the jury model using all the predictors. Let each of the 19 predictors see the original data, each make 19 separate decisions, and then take a vote across the decisions. By vote we mean just the simple majority vote: if 10 *or more* of the predictions declare $B = 1$ then that's our group decision. If 10 or more vote the other way then declare $B = 0$.

But just where does this method take us? Given that we know at least approximately the individual error rates for each of the rules A_i, we can examine a table of binomial (simple coin-tossing) outcomes to see what the prediction error rate would be for our majority voting method. An *error* in this majority voting scheme occurs when we know that $B = 0$ but 10 or more of the A_i state that $B = 1$. Thus, to evaluate our ensemble approach we are asking the statistical question "what is the probability that we find 11 or more heads coming up when we toss 19 coins, where the probability of any single head is 0.30, and the tosses are independent?"

Using the standard tables we find that the probability of making an error is 0.0326. Surely this is astonishing. Our jury scheme is doing remarkably well and uses only very weak juror members. Continuing, if the error rate for each predictor is 0.40, then using the majority vote scheme leads to an error rate of 0.1861, again a substantial improvement. Let's pause to restate and consider the implications of these simple calculations.

We see that our *if* predictors are approximately independent of each other, and *if* all are only weakly correlated individually with the outcome (that is, the separate error rates are rather high, being 0.30 or 0.40 for example), then by combining the separate predictors using the majority vote method, we make an error that is considerably less than the individual rate. This kind of calculation, and other more involved voting schemes, provide an important theoretical justification for the class of statistical learning methods called ensemble or committee methods.

Note next that we have said nothing about the individual juror members, the base classifiers in this scheme: details about how they each use the data are simply not required. Indeed, they could each be using the data in very different ways, effectively acting as technically unrelated statistical learning machines. In this sense our jurors are not communicating with each other. This is not standard in the usual juror system, but is essential for our ensemble approach.

Pushing this scheme still further, we see that the tables show that pooling decisions over increasingly large numbers of predictors continues to drive down the overall error rate, as long as the predictors continue to be independent.

Obtaining complete statistical independence from among many prediction schemes (juror members) is impractical, yet from among a very large list of candidate predictors (base classifiers), it may be possible to consider multiple subsets of them that are uncorrelated, one subset being approximately uncorrelated with or independent of any other subset. The idea here is that each predictor is given a different sector of the data by being assigned to make a decision using distinct subsets of features. Each subset of features can then be used as input to any machine learning system, and each subset can generate a single predictor. Subsequent pooling over the many predictions often then leads to the dramatic error reductions that we've just demonstrated under the strict independence assumption. How to select these relatively independent classifiers is then the new challenge problem. Using random selections of the data *and* random selections of subsets of features is one possibility: see Chapter 7 and the Random Forests method.

It's also true that when we can't drive down the correlations between the predictors then we can't expect to *automatically* generate a majority voting scheme with a greatly reduced error rate. The extreme example of this important point occurs when the separate predictors are clearly highly correlated with each other. Even without generating a simulated dataset or producing the required mathematics, we can see that in this case the separate predictors act approximately as a *single* prediction scheme, possibly each with poor error rates and so with essentially high error rate even when acting jointly.

Moreover, there is another situation that is more problematic. Consider, then, the case where we are given many really good predictors, and try to drive the error rate down still further. The extreme case occurs here with multiple predictors having basically zero error rates. But now in this seemingly good situation it is clear that the predictors must act almost always in concert: in order for each of them to routinely make the correct decision on the next case presented to the group, they must make the *same* decision on that next case, that is, they must make the same correct decision. This decision will be correct with high probability of course, but they will still be acting with high correlation. If all make the same (correct) decision then their predictions must be highly correlated between themselves: they cannot be statistically independent. Thus, it becomes increasingly difficult to prove that we can get large reductions in the error rate, using already very low error predictors, under *just* the assumption that they can act independently. More precisely, this underscores the fact that our binary outcomes are real-world decision-making rules and not simple, binomial coin-tossing mechanisms.

Informally summarizing, a crowd becomes a provably better decision scheme *if* every individual acts nearly, or, better still, completely independently of all the others, but should the individuals already be good predictors then a large, group error rate reduction is harder to achieve simply by taking averages. Extremely good predictors by definition can't act independently of each other.

12.3 Model averaging

There are other important theoretical results on ensemble methods that can be invoked to promote committee decision rules. We summarize some of them here.

(1) Pooling decision rules, possibly with weights estimated from the data or otherwise, can lead to *Bayesian model averaging*. Without going into the justification for using any Bayesian procedure (as opposed to a purely frequentist one; see Note 2), it is possible that combining many rules can lead to better performance, without invoking statistical independence among the rules. To verify that such improvements are possible usually requires limiting the class of rules (or models) from which we select in our final weighting scheme. The central idea here is that some models (rules) are more probable as truly representing the unobserved state of Nature than others, and the data can help us weight the various rules. This is still somewhat controversial, or perhaps impractical, as a principle of inference and decision-making, but its origins need not prevent it from leading to good decision rules and classification methods. Our earlier discussion on naïve Bayes learning machines made this point, and we have made it in other contexts apart from discussions of the Bayes paradigm: the efficiency of a learning machine need not be automatically understood or evaluated on the basis of its original, formal motivation.

(2) Pooling decision rules can also mean simply averaging the decisions made by a family of rules without a particular rationale for how the separate rules are generated, and without requiring statistical impendence. It can be demonstrated mathematically under quite general conditions, that quite primitive, individual (base) classifiers can eventually generate optimal rules, as the sample size increases. Indeed, this can happen even when the base classifiers are provably not optimal (are not Bayes consistent); see Section 2.11. In words, taking averages over many not-so-good base classifiers can lead to provably very good classifiers. There is some statistical and mathematical delicacy in this argument, in that a not-good base classifier can be rescued under certain circumstances and sometimes cannot be rescued; see, Biau and Devroye (2010), Biau *et al.* (2008, 2010b).

Typically to prove large-sample results for ensemble learning machines, the growth in the numbers of classifiers and the increase in the sample size both need to be monitored. If the numbers of classifiers are not allowed to grow, or if the data seen by each classifier is not increasing sufficiently fast, then all bets are off, so to speak. It is this crucial balance between data size

Table 12.1 The method of Mojirsheibani (1999, table 1) applied to a dataset with 10 data points and using three machines. To classify a test data point z, suppose the three machines applied to z yield output $\{1, 0, 1\}$. There are four occurrences of this triple decision by the machines, at training points #4, 6, 8, 10. Of these four points, three are associated with the outcome $y = 0$ (at #6, 8, 10) and one with the outcome $y = 1$ (at #4). The majority vote over these training data outcomes yields the prediction $z = 0$

| Data point # | Output for each machine | | | |
	M1	M2	M3	Outcome y
1	0	1	1	0
2	1	0	0	0
3	1	1	1	1
4	1	0	1	1
5	0	0	0	1
6	1	0	1	0
7	0	1	0	1
8	1	0	1	0
9	1	1	0	1
10	1	0	1	0

and ensemble size that has to be studied to determine the ultimate error rate of the method. Note that we have already seen the importance of this balancing act in determining the optimality of a single classifier: a k-nearest neighbor scheme is optimal (Bayes consistent) if k, the number of neighbors under consideration for any new data point, is allowed to grow as the sample grows, and do so at a certain rate. A fixed k won't provably lead to good decision-making.

(3) Finally we turn to a most interesting method for pooling machines; see Mojirsheibani (1999, 2002). In this scheme we start with any finite collection of classifiers. We don't need to know how any of them work and we don't specify the data to which we apply this method. The purely mechanical aspect of the method is shown in Table 12.1.

The voting process of the method is very similar to that of a single decision tree, where the terminal node for a test data point is inspected and a local vote taken. For three machines there will always be $2 \times 2 \times 2 = 8$ terminal nodes, and the order in which we process the three outcomes for a test point is immaterial. So far, simple enough.

Here is the amazing property of this scheme: it can be shown to be Bayes consistent with large samples, as the number of machines increases, and the method is always at least as good as the best machine in the collection (in a certain carefully stated probabilistic sense). Thus, if just one of the machines happens to be Bayes consistent, the whole scheme is also Bayes consistent, and, indeed we don't need to know which of the three is the Bayes machine. Moreover, in the absence of having any Bayes consistent machine in the collection, the procedure is *still* itself Bayes consistent for large samples.

As with any tree-like system we need to be sure the occupancy rates of the terminal nodes are sufficiently large, and the number of machines needs to grow as well, but not too fast. The rate is spelled out in Mojirsheibani (1999), and closely resembles those derived in DGL for other provably optimal classes of machines, as just described above. From practical experience Mojirsheibani reports that as long as the number M of machines is in the range

$$2 < M < \log n$$

where n is the sample size, then one should expect good results.

Two things are important to note about this method. First, it is not a committee method: we're not voting across the decisions of many machines, but voting locally in terminal nodes as directed by the machines. In a sense, the "committee" here is the population in the terminal node in which the test data point ends up. Second, any correlation between the machines need not be examined or accounted for. Some of the machines could be close cousins mathematically (all forms of support vector machines, say, with different kernels), and others completely unrelated. Kinship is irrelevant.

Using this scheme thus partially obviates any need to choose from a collection of machines: use all of them, with the expectation that the best machine in the lot will be improved upon without our having to decide which machine that might be, and if there isn't any very good machine in the lot, the scheme is still large-sample optimal. Mojirsheibani (1999) has several explanatory data examples, some of which do contain a very good, single classifier and some of which don't.

Notes

(1) For an elegant and insightful discussion of Condorcet's Jury Theorem – dating from 1785! – and many other aspects of decision-making generally, see Körner (2008), Saari (2008), Gintis (2009).

(2) This is a furiously developing topic with numerous vocal adherents. See, for example, http://www2.research.att.com/~volinsky/bma.html.

Summary and conclusions

I wake to sleep, and take my waking slow.
I feel my fate in what I cannot fear.
I learn by going where I have to go.

Theodore Roethke[1]

13.1 Where have we been?

The world of learning machines continues to grow rapidly, expand out in novel directions, and extend the search for explanations of previous successes. We have seen that there are previously hidden links between machines that are being uncovered, and alternative versions of machines that markedly improve on earlier ones. The subject is far from being a mature technology. Our discussion of learning machines is, therefore, only a narrowly developed snapshot of what is known and available at the time of writing (Summer 2010). Yet some broad conclusions are nonetheless clear. And we discuss several kinds of interesting machines that are of very recent vintage, or, should be invented right away.

Statistical learning machines are computer-intensive schemes that allow the researcher to venture into data realms where most of the classical statistical assumptions no longer apply. They are often massively nonparametric, highly nonlinear, and yet benefit from fine-tuning when applied to specific datasets. Since the machines don't depend on familiar distributional assumptions of the data – which need not be multivariate normal, for example – the results from theory showing how well they can perform are

[1] "The Waking," © 1953 by Theodore Roethke, from *Collected Poems of Theodore Roethke* by Theodore Roethke. Used by permission of Doubleday, a division of Random House, Inc. and Faber and Faber, Ltd.

necessarily deep and nontrivial technical results. This theory could be out-lined only briefly in Section 2.11. Yet we encourage the reader to press forward into this mathematical thicket, this probabilistic forest, as far as time and patience will allow. For the venturesome there are stunning vistas, gleaming rewards.

More recently revealed among such rewards is the connection between local and global information. Let's review this connection. At several places in previous chapters, we asserted a generalization about information-gathering: all information is local and collective, only rarely global and singular. This generalization can be made very precise. Indeed, theory reveals that *all* good prediction and classification methods – those that are Bayes consistent for all possible distributions of the data – must be *local*. That is, only data near the point to be classified (or upon which a prediction is made) are needed for making the classification or prediction; see Section 2.11. And as more data is collected the size of this small neighborhood about any new test data point should shrink to zero. As might be expected where mathe-matical theory is involved, there are varying senses of *local* in the technical literature, including one in which data far from the given point can be mutated (a lot, a little) without changing the prediction for a test point, but the idea remains the same.

Closely related to locality is this: all good procedures must correctly see at least one of the global features of the data, and in only a very weak sense. One version of the finding is this: the good procedure needs on average to only predict the correct mean of all the outcomes, the dependent values in the regression setting for example.

Another less intuitive but important insight driven by this study of local and global properties is that machines that seem to be quite nonlocal, and support vector machines and boosting methods for two very surprising examples, are indeed local as can be defined above. But the starting points, the essential algorithmic definitions of these important machines, give no indication of this locality. Something like this might have been anticipated, since our task is to make classifications for *any* given distribution and this means a successful machine must surely apprehend – come to well understand – the local behavior of the data at hand.

Most good methods do eventually make the right decision: given enough data, with at least some signal present, they make decisions that are very close to Bayes optimal. But as we warned in Chapter 2, even the best methods may approach the golden endpoint very slowly, and the rate depends crucially on the structure of the data being presented to it.

Let's next review how machines can be collected and evaluated.

13.2 So many machines

Most learning machines require some form of tuning, some – often limited – degree of adjustment by the user, given the data under study. In our experience this tuning is important to pursue, but good schemes make this fairly easy. It is also our experience that there is little gained by obsessive finely graded tuning. Instead, once some modest tuning is completed a much more important problem arises, that of evaluating the performance of the machine. We devoted Chapter 11 to this problem, and declared that most of our energy and brainpower allocated for analysis of data should be directed toward this evaluation.

A closely related problem is the careful comparison of one machine with another, and this is important for two reasons.

First, if the data has any signal at all then most machines will detect it. We invoke the Rosetta Stone principle: if Nature is trying to tell us anything she will say the same thing in at least three languages. So the real question is, are any of these machines arguably better than the others for my data? The Agresti–Tango methods (Chapter 11) for pairwise comparisons of machines are well suited for this task. Other refinements of this paired-comparison problem continue to be developed, but the basic idea is the same: each pair of machines needs to be studied on how it predicts (classifies) a subject and the results need to account for the correlation between the predictions. The data-analytic epoch, when simple estimated mean values of error rates (however accurate) can suffice for statements about performance, is long gone.

Second, we freely admit that many machines studied in this text are somewhat mysterious, though powerful engines. Even recent literature on the theory side of machine learning highlights the fact that *why* certain machines do so well is still a matter of discussion; see the long, multithreaded discussion in Mease and Wyner (2008) (with extended Comments and Rejoinder). But as a more urgent practical matter, even a single classification tree can be hard to interpret, especially since the top levels of any tree need not be at all informative about the importance of one feature compared with another; see Chapter 6. A robust, generally excellent method such as Random Forests, which grow and aggregate thousands of trees, is even more opaque. As discussed in Chapter 6, even single trees can be misread and seemingly different trees can comprise the same partitions of the data separately.

Thus simpler, usually small and linear models can be invoked, once the machine has asserted that good predictive information is available in the data. But to replace one cabinet of curiosities, a black box, with a simple, open book (or, model) requires two things: first, that the performance of the small model is as least as good as the cabinet, and second, that the features used in the small model are representative of the often vastly larger collection of features used in the machine.

We discussed both problems in Chapter 11. And we also alerted the researcher to the problem that one list of good features may be very different from another equally good list. Indeed, we argued that finding multiple good lists might be a more productive and more robust path to scientific discovery. Closely related to the problem of finding good predictors is the usual instability of any such lists. The preference problem, as discussed in Chapter 9, perhaps has no perfect solution (but see the recent work of Melnik *et al.*, 2007), and as shown there, under very plausible conditions, provably has no unique solution. We think Nature is trying to tell us something. Now where did we store that Rosetta Stone …

We also discussed that, having found a few good, or even a collection of only modestly good, machines for some data, there is still another option available that makes the identification of a single, winning machine probably unnecessary. That is, ensembles or committees of machines can often improve on members of the committee. To see this we started, in Chapter 9, with Condorcet's Jury Theorem, 1785! – we do so love highlighting that date – and discussed more recent developments. One such recent finding is that inconsistent machines (those provably not Bayes consistent) can be collected together into ensembles that are Bayes consistent; see Biau *et al.* (2010b). And one earlier, equally impressive result is that weak learners can be collected together and boosted, using a scheme that successively, jointly adjusts weights for the machines and the data; see Chapter 3. The modified committee method of Mojirsheibani (1999) is equally impressive: if a good machine lurks buried in our list of machines, this combining method will be at least as good as that one, even when we don't know which of the machines is the good one.

13.3 Binary decision or probability estimate?

There has been another recurrent theme in our work: do we want to solve the pure classification problem *or* the probability of group membership problem? More sharply still, *can* we solve the probability of membership problem? We have seen that a good solution for the latter problem, a good probability estimate, is more informative, and then necessarily generates a good classification for the binary problem of putting a subject in one group or another. But these probability solutions are also harder to derive, and much harder to validate. Indeed, we spent some time in Chapter 5 on the calibration problem for logistic regression, without coming to very satisfying results (but we did display goodness-of-fit methods collected and studied by Kuss, 2002 that work for logistic regression models).

And it's not currently known if a very good group classification method will necessarily generate a good estimate of group probability. And it is not clear when a provably very good binary classifier can be converted into a probability estimator. This remains an important area of research. See Mease *et al.* (2007) for a necessary and cautionary story of the distinction between classification and probability estimation, and our discussion at the end of Chapter 2.

13.4 Survival machines? Risk machines?

Closely related to probability machines are two other approaches that we have also not discussed in this book, which deserve a book-length treatment in themselves. These are *survival machines*, which when presented with a syndrome or diagnosis then generate estimates of survival time: five-year survival after a course of treatment for breast cancer. Such machines start from biomedical, genetic and clinical information, and would parallel classical statistical models that have a long and rich pedigree; see, for example, Lawless and Yuan (2010). We note that Random Forests has an excellent

Survival Forest version, but we have not studied it in this text; see Ishwaran *et al.* (2008, 2010) and Omurlu *et al.* (2009).

Still another topic omitted from our discussion is the construction of a machine for *attributable risk estimation*. This is more interventional in nature, since the machine (model) is used to assess how changing biomedical circumstances might change the survival rate for a subject: does lowering trans fat intake by X% lead to a Y% increase in 10-year survival, holding all other factors fixed?

13.5 And where are we going?

Still other important topics omitted from our discussion include the following.

(a) *Longitudinal or repeated measures data.* These are well studied in classical statistics, but seem nearly invisible in the learning machine literature at present. Data with a time course – dynamic data – is central to biology and its machine analysis should be a subject of intense study and invention. Sequential time-series prediction using learning machines data has been considered here: Biau *et al.* (2010a).

(b) *Matched-case control data.* This could be investigated once we had a good probability machine. That is, given an estimate for the conditional probability of a pair, a prediction could follow much as it does in classical logistic regression, for which see chapter 9 in Agresti (1996).

(c) *Image classification, infinitely many features.* We have considered feature lists that can number in the thousands, and as we write (Summer 2010) we are systematically and successfully analyzing multiple, genome-wide datasets having 2.1 million features (SNPs). Classification problems for images – MRI brain scans, EKG or EEG plots, fingerprints, speech recording, spectra – and more generally classification of functions have effectively an *infinitely* long list of potential features. It is known that converging to the best possible prediction error rate is not at all certain using methods we have discussed so far. Instead newer methods, and some added restrictions on the "infinite" data are required; see, for example, Biau *et al.* (2010c), Berlinet *et al.* (2008).

(d) *Detection of anomalies, explanation of tiny details.* This is the problem opposite to placing a subject in the most plausible group: finding the unusual and unlikely in the data wherever it occurs; see, for example, the PhD thesis of Terran Lane (Lane, 2000) and Meinshausen (2006). Often, anomalous or hard-to-detect events are the most telling in terms of hidden structure: the very slight precession of the perihelion of Mercury was not predicted accurately by Newtonian mechanics (1687) but through the vastly more comprehensive analysis of Einstein's general relativity (1915). Another example of this process, which can be called *learning from error*, or, *discrepancy*, is given by retracing the discovery of argon in 1895, leading to the Nobel Prize for Rayleigh and Ramsay in 1906; see also Spanos (2010).

(e) *Cluster detection in the subjects.* The Random Forests and Random Jungles learning machines both have a built-in subject–subject clustering scheme, using MDS plots as we discussed in Chapter 2. Indeed the variable importance measures in each scheme can lead to refined prediction and clustering, since we could expect that distinct subgroups of patients have distinct lists of important features. More systematic use of forest and jungle clustering is highly recommended; see for example Shi *et al.* (2005).

(f) *Cluster detection in the features; small networks and cliques.* Just above we talked about starting with one machine and moving to a smaller one, a classical statistical procedure such as linear or logistic regression. Much is known about these classical methods and yet they can still provide surprises, where these surprises may arise when we try to transport the findings of the big machine to the small parametric model setting. We discussed this problem in Chapters 5, 8 and 9, but it bears continuous, close scrutiny: small sets of features that are active (important) in a machine are often jointly helping to make the prediction, where this entangled cooperation can be quite complex, and each of the features in the set may be a very weak predictor by itself. This is true, of course, for linear or logistic regression models, but some version of interaction in the classical models is often introduced directly into the model to account for this behavior. However, we have noted that apart from very simple constructions (products of two of the features, say), interaction is a not well-defined, perhaps indefinable term. Indeed, standard definitions of interaction, such as the product of two predictors, may be quite good, or not so good: recall the example of logistic regression on the cholesterol data in Chapter 5.

Next to the development of probability machines, this problem of network revelation – motif naming – is perhaps of most importance for biological research. Once we confidently declare signal as present in the data, then network detection, clique hunting, and module stamping become essential: see, for example, Biau and Bleakley (2006), Bleakley *et al.* (2007), and Lippert *et al.* (2009).

And this leads directly to the rapidly developing topic of *systems biology*, a subject for another time:

"So, Larry, tell me about networks and pathways ..."
"Signaling or metabolic?"

Appendix

A1:   Software used in this book

A2:   Data used in this book

A1: Software used in this book

Classification and Regression Tree; CART

We used the Matlab functions `treefit` and `treeval` for learning and prediction, respectively. We use Gini's diversity index as our splitting criterion. But see also Note 1(c) at the end of Chapter 7.

k-Nearest Neighbor; k-NN

k-NN algorithms are relatively simple to implement, but the best are truly fast implementations. We used several implementations and list two that are available at Matlab Central: an implementation by Yi Cao (at Cranfield University on 25 March 2008) called *Efficient K-Nearest Neighbor Search using JIT* http://www.mathworks.com/matlabcentral/fileexchange/19345-efficient-k-nearest-neighbor-search-using-jit and an implementation by Luigi Giaccari called *Fast k-Nearest Neighbors Search* http://www.math works.es/matlabcentral/fileexchange/22190.

Support Vector Machines; SVM

We used the implementation SVM*light* that can be found at http://svmlight.joachims.org/.

A number of other software packages for SVMs can be found at http://www.support-vector-machines.org/SVM_soft.html.

Fisher Linear Discriminant Analysis; LDA

Matlab code for performing Fisher LDA is provided below.

Logistic Regression

Matlab code for performing logistic regression is provided below.

Neural Networks

Neural Networks is a broad term that includes a number of related implementations. In this book we used one that optimizes the number of nodes in the hidden layers. This is derived from work by Broyden–Fletcher–Goldfarb–Shanno (*BFGS*) and by DJC MacKay; see MacKay (1992a,b).

The implementation we used was written for Matlab by Sigurdur Sigurdsson (2002) and is based on an older neural classifier written by Morten with Pedersen. It is available in the ANN:DTU Toolbox http://isp.imm.dtu.dk/toolbox/ann/index.html.

As stated on that website, all code can be used freely in research and other nonprofit applications. If you publish results obtained with the ANN:DTU Toolbox you are asked to cite the relevant sources.

Multiple neural network packages are available for R (search "neural network" at http://cran.r-project.org/.

Still other free packages for neural network classification (NuMap and NuClass, available only for Windows) can be found at http://www-ee.uta.edu/eeweb/IP/Software/Software.htm.

A convenient place to find a collection of Matlab implementations is "Matlab Central" http://www.mathworks.com/matlabcentral/.

For example, Neural Network Classifiers written by Sebastien Paris is available at http://www.mathworks.com/matlabcentral/fileexchange/17415.

A commercial package "Neural Network Toolbox" is also available for Matlab.

Boosting

We used BoosTexter, available at http://www.cs.princeton.edu/~schapire/boostexter.html.

For this implementation see Schapire and Singer (2000). As stated on the home page above, "the object code for BoosTexter is available free from AT&T for non-commercial research or educational purposes."

Random Forests; RF

Random Forests (written for R) can be obtained from http://cran.r-project.org/web/packages/randomForest/index.html.

SAS® programs

Logistic regressions for stroke study analysis were done in SAS® version 9.1.3 PROC LOGISTIC.

Custom SAS® version 8.2 PROC IML code, macro %GOFLOGIT written by Oliver Kuss (2002), was used for model goodness-of-fit analysis in logistic regression.

R code for comparison of correlated error estimates

We applied an adjusted Wald confidence interval and the Tango score interval, using the R code as described in Agresti and Min (2005).

Matlab code

Code for **Fisher Linear Discriminant Analysis**: fLDA.m

```
function [ConfMatrix,decisions,prms]=fLDA(LearnSamples, ...
LearnLabels,TestSamples,TestLabels)
% Usage:
% ConfMatrix,decisions,prms]=fLDA(LearnSamples,LearnLabels,
% TestSamples,TestLabels)
%
% The code expects that the LearnSamples and TestSamples be
% n x m matrices where n is the number of the cases (samples)
% and each row contains the m-predictor values for each case.
% Otherwise, transpose the data, i.e. uncomment the lines below:
% LearnSamples=LearnSamples';
% TestSamples=TestSamples';

% separate the data into "positives" and "negatives"
ipos=find(LearnLabels==1);
ineg=find(LearnLabels==0);
predpos=LearnSamples(ipos,:);
predneg=LearnSamples(ineg,:);
nsamp_pos=length(predpos);
nsamp_neg=length(predneg);

% obtain the covariance matrix and the means for "positives" and
% "negatives"
[Spos, meanpos]=getSmat(predpos);
[Sneg, meanneg]=getSmat(predneg);
```

```
% obtain Fisher LDA projection wproj that maximizes J(w)
wproj=inv(Spos+Sneg)*(meanpos-meanneg)';
wproj=wproj/norm(wproj)

% find appropriate decision threshold
sp=sqrt(trace(Spos)/nsamp_pos);
sm=sqrt(trace(Sneg)/nsamp_neg);
mnsm=(sm*meanpos+sp*meanneg)/(sm+sp);
cthresh=mnsm*wproj;

if nargout>2 % if asking for it, provide the parameters of fLDA
 prms={wproj,cthresh,mnsm};
end

decisions=[];
ConfMatrix=[];
if nargin>2 % if testsamples provided
 % run the discriminant on the testing data
 cpred=TestSamples*wproj;
 decisions=(cpred>cthresh)';
 if nargin>3 % if testlabels provided
  % obtain the confusion matrix (1 indicates that we
  % want the raw counts)
  ConfMatrix=GetConfTable(decisions,TestLabels,1);
 end
end

% Supporting functions
% get a covariance matrix of x
function [Smat,meanx]=getSmat(x)
 meanx=mean(x);
 zmn=x-repmat(meanx,size(x,1),1);
 Smat=zmn'*zmn;

% get a confusion matrix
function [ConfTable,labls]=GetConfTable(FinalDecision,...
        TestLabels,counts)
% function [ConfTable,labls]=GetConfTable(FinalDecision,
% TestLabels,counts)
% Returns confusion table based on the machine decisions
% (FinalDecision) and the known outcomes.
```

```
% If the flag counts=0 returns confusion matrix in terms
% of fractions (percentages), otherwise returns confusion
% matrix as raw counts

if nargin<3, counts=0;, end
% labls=fliplr(flipud(unique(TestLabels)));
 labls=fliplr(unique(TestLabels));
 nlabls=length(labls);
 if nlabls == 1 % if all decisions were the same
  nlabls=2;
  if labls(1), labls=[labls(1),0]; else labls=[1,0]; end
 end
 ConfTable=zeros(nlabls);
 for ilb=1:nlabls
  i1=find(TestLabels==labls(ilb));
  for jlb=1:nlabls
   i2=find(FinalDecision(i1)==labls(jlb));
   if counts
     ConfTable(jlb,ilb)=length(i2);
   else
     ConfTable(jlb,ilb)=length(i2)/length(i1);
   end
  end
 end
```

Code for **Logistic Regression**: logisticr.m

```
function lrresult = logisticr(LRSamples, LRinp, fitit, wts)
% function lrresult = logisticr(LRSamples, LRinp, fitit, wts)
% parameter fitit determines if fitting or evaluation is used
% for fitit=1:
%  input: LearnSamples as LRSampls and LearnLabels as LRinp
%  returns LR model (npredictors+1) parameters in lrresults
% for fitit=0 or fitit=2:
%  input: TestingSamples (LRSamples), LR parameters (LRinp)
%  returns probabilites (fitit=0) or
%  log-odds (fitit=2) in lrresults
%
% Example: (using decision threshold "logisticthreshold"):
% lrprms=mylogistic(LearnSamples, LearnLabels, 1);
```

```
% decisions=mylogistic(TestSamples,lrprms) > logisticthreshold;
% ConfMatrix=GetConfTable(decisions,TestLabels);

if nargin<3 fitit=0; end

switch fitit
 case {0,2} % return the LR values
  [nsamps, mpred] = size(LRSamples);
  inputmat=[LRSamples,ones(nsamps,1)];
  liny = inputmat * LRinp;
  if fitit==2
   lrresult = liny
  else
   lrresult = invlogit(liny);
  end
 case 1 % Obtain LR parameters (fitting)
 % specify desired precision and maximal number of
 % Newton-Ralphson iterations, trade precision (small itereps,
 % e.g. 1e-12) for speed (larger itereps, e.g. 1e-7)
  itereps = 1e-9;
  maxiter = 100;
  [nsamps, mpred] = size(LRSamples)
  inputmat=[LRSamples,ones(nsamps,1)];
  mprms=mpred+1;

  % assume all weights equal, in not specified
  if nargin < 4, wts = ones(nsamps,1); end

  % initialize iterations
  lrresult=zeros(mprms,1);
  lrnlabels=LRinp';
  prevexpy=-ones(size(lrnlabels));
  for iter=1:maxiter
   liny=inputmat*lrresult;
   expy=invlogit(liny);
   % LR weights based on derivative of invlogit (=p(1-p))
   lrw=max(5*eps, expy.*(1-expy)); % avoiding zero lrw for
   liny=liny+(lrnlabels-expy)./lrw; % update with W^(-1)(y-p)
   % adjust prescribed weights "wts" with LR weights to
   % obtain the final weights matrix
   weights=spdiags(lrw.*wts, 0, nsamps, nsamps);
```

```
% can then be obtained as equiv. linear regression
% to modifed liny
lrresult=inv(inputmat'*weights*inputmat) ...
    *inputmat'*weights* liny;
 if sum(abs(expy-prevexpy)) < nsamps*itereps
  break;
 end
 prevexpy=expy;
 end
otherwise
 disp(sprintf('The value fitit=%d not implemented yet', fitit))
end

function logodds=logit(p)
 logodds=log(p./(1-p));

function p=invlogit(lodds)
 p=1./(1+exp(-lodds));
```

A2: Data used in this book

We principally used three datasets: (1) the German stroke dataset, (2) the lupus dataset, and (3) the simulated cholesterol data. These are all discussed in Chapter 4. Unfortunately, neither the German nor the lupus data are available for public use. As a nice alternative we suggest accessing the thoroughly edited and maintained data collection at the University of California (Irvine) machine learning website: http://archive.ics.uci.edu/ml/.

As of Spring 2010, there are nearly 200 datasets available, providing ground material for the study of nearly every aspect of machine learning, and derived from an astonishing range of subjects.

One caution, however, as we discussed in Section 2.10: that is, the benchmarking problem raised by using data to declare single winners. This is indeed a problem since for any given dataset on which a given scheme does best among a set of schemes, there is a counter dataset and an alternative scheme such that the alternative scheme can be selected to be Bayes consistent, and do better than the original "winning" scheme at every sample size.

Moreover, as discussed in Chapter 12, for any finite collection of machines there is an ensemble machine that does at least as well as the best in that collection. Which is to say that declaring a single winner in a machine arms race is a misdirected use of computing resources and brain power.

References

Adami, C (2006). Reducible complexity. *Science*, **312**: 61–3.

Agarwal, S, P Niyogi (2009). Generalization bounds for ranking algorithms via algorithmic stability. *Journal of Machine Learning Research*, **10**: 441–74.

Agresti, A (1996). *An Introduction to Categorical Data Analysis*. John Wiley & Sons.

Agresti, A, C Franklin (2009). *Statistics: The Art and Science of Learning from Data*. Second Edition. Prentice-Hall.

Agresti, A, Y Min (2005). Simple improved confidence intervals for comparing matched proportions. *Statistics in Medicine*, **24**: 729–40.

Ailon, N, M Mohri (2008). An efficient reduction of ranking to classification. In *Proceedings of the 21st Annual Conference on Learning Theory*.

Alqallaf, FA, KP Konis, RD Martin, RH Zamar (2002). Scalable robust covariance and correlation estimates for data mining. Proceedings of the SIGKDD Conference 2002, Edmonton, Alberta, Canada: 1–10.

Anderson-Sprecher, R (1994). Model comparisons and R^2. *American Statistician*, **48**(2): 113–17.

Archer, KJ, VR Mas (2009). Ordinal response prediction using bootstrap aggregation, with application to a high-throughput methylation dataset. *Statistics in Medicine*, in press.

Banzhaf, W, G Beslon, S Christensen, JA Foster, F Képès, V Lefort, JF Miller, M Radman, JJ Ramsden (2006). From artificial evolution to computational evolution: a research agenda. *Nature Reviews Genetics*, **7**: 729–35.

Bartlett, PL *et al.* (2004). Discussion of three boosting papers. *Annals of Statistics*, **32**(1): 85–134.

Berger, JO, RL Wolpert (1988). *The Likelihood Principle*. Institute of Mathematical Statistics, Lecture Notes – Monograph Series, Vol. 6.

Berk, RA (2008). *Statistical Learning from a Regression Perspective*. Springer-Verlag.

Berlinet, A, G Biau, L Rouvière (2008). Functional supervised classification with wavelets. *Annales de l'ISUP*, **52**: 61–80.

Biau, G (2010). Analysis of a random forests model. Submitted to *Journal of Machine Learning Research*.

Biau, G and K Bleakley (2006). Statistical inference on graphs. *Statistics & Decisions*, **24**: 209–32.

Biau, G, K Bleakley, L Györfi, G Ottucsák (2010a). Nonparametric sequential prediction of time series. *Journal of Nonparametric Statistics*, **22**: 297–317.

Biau, G, F Cérou, A Guyader (2010b). On the rate of convergence of the bagged nearest neighbor estimate. *Journal of Machine Learning Research*, **11**: 687–712.

Biau, G, F Cérou, A Guyader (2010c). Rates of convergence of the functional *k*-nearest neighbor estimate. *IEEE Transactions on Information Theory*, **56**: 2034–40.

Biau, G, L Devroye (2005). Density estimation by the penalized combinatorial method. *Journal of Multivariate Analysis*, **94**: 196–208.

Biau, G, L Devroye (2010). On the layered nearest neighbor estimate, the bagged nearest neighbor estimate and the random forest method in regression and classification. *Journal of Multivariate Analysis*, in press.

Biau, G, L Devroye, G Lugosi (2008). Consistency of random forests and other averaging classifiers. *Journal of Machine Learning Research*, **9**: 2015–33.

Blanchard, G, G Lugosi, N Vayatis (2003). On the rate of convergence of regularized boosting methods. *Journal of Machine Learning Research* **4**: 861–94.

Bleakley, K, G Biau, J-P Vert (2007). Supervised reconstruction of biological networks with local models. *Bioinformatics*, **23**: 157–65.

Bonita, R, R Beaglehole (1988). Recovery of motor function after stroke. *Stroke*, **19**: 1497–500.

Borg, I, PJF Groenen (2005). *Modern Multidimensional Scaling*. Second Edition. Springer-Verlag.

Bossuyt, PM, L Irwig, J Craig, P Glasziou (2006). Comparative accuracy: assessing new tests against existing diagnostic pathways. *British Medical Journal*, **332**: 1089–92.

Breiman, L (2004). The 2002 Wald Memorial Lectures. Population theory for boosting ensembles. *Annals of Statistics*, **32**(1): 1–11.

Breiman, L, J Friedman, CJ Stone, RA Olshen (1984, 1993). *Classification and Regression Trees*. Chapman & Hall.

Carlin, BP, TA Louis (2000). *Bayes and Empirical Bayes Methods for Data Analysis*. Second Edition. Chapman & Hall/CRC Press.

Casale, S, A Russo, G Scebba, S Serrano (2008). Speech Emotion Classification Using Machine Learning Algorithms. 2008 *IEEE International Conference on Semantic Computing*: 158–65.

Claeskens, G, NL Hjort (2008). *Model Selection and Model Averaging*. Cambridge University Press.

Cover, T, P Hart (1967). Nearest neighbor pattern classification. *IEEE Transactions on Information Theory*, **13**: 21–7.

Cox, DR (1958). Two further applications of a model for binary regression. *Biometrika*, **45**: 562–5.

Cox, TF, MAA Cox (2001). *Multidimensional Scaling*. Second Edition. Springer-Verlag.

Cristianini, N, J Shawe-Taylor (2000). *Support Vector Machines, and Other Kernel-Based Learning Methods*. Cambridge University Press.

Davison, AC, DV Hinkley (1997). *Bootstrap Methods and their Application*. Cambridge University Press.

Devroye, L, L Györfi, G Lugosi (1996). *A Probabilistic Theory of Pattern Recognition*. Springer-Verlag.

Devroye, L, G Lugosi (2001). *Combinatorial Methods in Density Estimation*. Springer-Verlag.

Devroye, L, T Wagner (1976). A distribution-free performance bound in error estimation. *IEEE Transactions on Information Theory*, **22**: 586–7.

Díaz-Uriarte, R, S Alvarez de Andrés (2006). Gene selection and classification of microarray data using random forest. *BMC Bioinformatics 2006*, **7**:3 doi:10.1186/1471-2105-7-3.

Draper, NR (1984). The Box–Wetz criterion versus R^2. *Journal of the Royal Statistical Society*, Series A (General), **147**(1): 100–103.

Draper, NR, H Smith (1998). *Applied Regression Analysis*. John Wiley & Sons.

Edgington, ES (1995). *Randomization Tests*. Third Edition. Marcel-Dekker.

Efron, B, R Tibshirani (1997). Improvement on cross-validation: the 632+ bootstrap method. *Journal of the American Statistical Association*, **92**: 548–60.

Elashoff, JD, RM Elashoff, GE Goldman (1967). On the choice of variables in classification problems with dichotomous variables. *Biometrika*, **54**: 668–70.

Fagin, R, R Kumar, D Sivakumar (2003). Comparing top k lists. *SIAM Journal of Discrete Mathematics*, **20**(3): 628–48.

Fagin, R, R Kumar, M Mahdian, S Sivakumar, E Vee (2006). Comparing partial rankings. *SIAM Journal of Discrete Mathematics*, **20**(3): 628–48.

Forti, A, GL Foresti (2006). Growing hierarchical tree SOM: an unsupervised neural network with dynamic topology. *Neural Networks*, **19**(10): 1568–80.

Freedman, D (1991). Statistical models and shoe leather. *Sociological Methodology*, **21**: 291–313.

Freedman D (1995). Some issues in the foundation of statistics. *Foundations of Science*, **1**: 19–39.

Freedman, D (1997). From association to causation via regression. *Advances in Applied Mathematics*, **18**: 59–110.

Freedman, D (1999). From association to causation: some remarks on the history of statistics. *Statistical Science*, **14**(3): 243–58.

Freedman, D (2009). *Statistical Models: Theory and Practice*. Revised Edition. Cambridge University Press.

Garcia-Pedrajas, N, D Ortiz-Boyer (2008). Boosting random subspace method. *Neural Networks*, **21**: 1344–62.

Gelman, A, JB Carlin, HS Stern, DB Rubin (2004). *Bayesian Data Analysis*. Second Edition. Chapman & Hall/CRC Press.

Getoor, L, B Taskar (eds) (2007). *Introduction to Statistical Relational Learning*. MIT Press.

Ghosh, D, AM Chinnaiyan (2005). Classification and selection of biomarkers in genomic data using LASSO. *Journal of Biomedicine and Biotechnology*, **2**: 147–54.

Gintis, H (2009). *The Bounds of Reason: Game Theory and the Unification of the Behavioural Sciences*. Princeton University Press.

Glantz, SA (2002). *Primer of Biostatistics*. Sixth Edition. McGraw-Hill.

Gneiting, T, AE Raftery (2007). Strictly proper scoring rules, prediction, and estimation. *Journal of the American Statistical Association*, **102**(477): 359–78.

Good, P (2005). *Permutation, Parametric, and Bootstrap Tests of Hypotheses*. Third Edition. Springer-Verlag.

Guyatt, GH *et al.* (1992). Evidence-based medicine. *Journal of the American Medical Association*, **268**(17): 2420–25.

Györfi, L, M Kohler, A Krzyżak, H Walk (2002, 2010). *A Distribution-Free Theory of Nonparametric Regression.* Springer-Verlag.

Hamedani, GG, HW Volkmer (2009). Letter to the Editor. *American Statistician,* **63**(3): 295.

Hand, DJ (1997). *Construction and Assessment of Classification Rules.* John Wiley & Sons.

Hand, DJ (2006). Classifier technology and the illusion of progress (with Comments and Rejoinder). *Statistical Science,* **21**(1): 1–34.

Hardin, J, A Mitani, L Hicks, B VanKoten (2007). A robust measure of correlation between two genes on a microarray. *BMC Bioinformatics,* **8**: 220–33.

Harrell, FE, Jr. (2001). *Regression Modeling Strategies.* Springer-Verlag.

Hastie, T, R Tibshirani, J Friedman (2009). *Elements of Statistical Learning.* Second Edition. Springer-Verlag.

Haunsperger, DB (1992). Dictionaries of paradoxes for statistical tests on k samples. *Journal of the American Statistical Association,* **87**(417): 149–55.

Haunsperger, DB (2003). Aggregated statistical rankings are arbitrary. *Social Choice and Welfare,* **20**: 261–72.

Haunsperger, DB, DG Saari (1991). The lack of consistency for statistical decision problems. *The American Statistician,* **45**(3): 252–5.

Healy, MJR (1984). The use of R^2 as a measure of goodness of fit. *Journal of the Royal Statistical Society,* Series A, **147**(4): 608–9.

Hilbe, JM (2009). *Logistic Regression Models.* Chapman & Hall/CRC Press.

Hilden, J (2003). Book review: Giovanni Parmigiani (2002). *Modeling in Medical Decision Making. A Bayesian Approach.* John Wiley & Sons. Published in *Statistics in Medicine,* **23**: 663–4.

Hilden, J (2004). Evaluation of diagnostic tests – the schism. (Notes on ROC methods and the value of information approach.) Available at: http://staff.pubhealth.ku.dk/~jh/.

Ho, TK (1998). The random subspace method for constructing decision forests. *IEEE Transactions on Pattern Analysis and Machine Intelligence,* **20**(8): 832–44.

Holden, ZA, M Crimmins, C Luce, EK Heyerdahl, P Morgan (2008). Analysis of Climate and Topographic Controls on Burn Severity in the Western United States (1984–2005), American Geophysical Union, Fall Meeting 2008, abstract #GC21A-0708.

Hosmer, DW Jr, S Lemeshow (2000). *Applied Logistic Regression.* Second Edition. John Wiley & Sons.

Hothorn, T, K Hornik, A Zeileis (2006). Unbiased recursive partitioning: a conditional inference framework. *Journal of Computational and Graphical Statistics,* **15**: 651–74.

Hu, B, M Palta, J Shao (2006). Properties of R^2 statistics for logistic regression. *Statistics in Medicine,* **25**: 1383–95.

Ingsrisawang, L, S Ingsriswang, S Somchit, P Aungsuratana, W Khantiyanan (2008). Machine Learning Techniques for Short-Term Rain Forecasting System in the Northeastern Part of Thailand. *Proceedings of the World Academy of Science, Engineering and Technology,* **31** July: 248–53.

Ishwaran, H, LF James, M Zarepour (2009). An alternative to the m out of n bootstrap. *Journal of Statistical Planning and Inference,* **139**: 788–801.

Ishwaran, H, UB Kogalur, EH Blackstone, MS Lauer (2008). Random survival forests. *The Annals of Applied Statistics*, **2**(3): 841–60.

Ishwaran, H, UB Kogalur, EZ Gorodeski, AJ Minn, MS Lauer (2010). High-dimensional variable selection for survival data. *Journal of the American Statistical Association*, **105**(489): 205–17.

Japkowicz, N (2009). Bibliography for imbalanced (unbalanced) data analysis. http://www. site.uottawa.ca/~nat/Research/class_imbalance_bibli.html.

Jerebko, AK, JD Malley, M Franaszek, RM Summers (2003). Multiple neural network classification scheme for detection of colonic polyps in CT colonography data sets. *Academic Radiology*, **10**: 154–60.

Jerebko, AK, JD Malley, M Franaszek, RM Summers (2005). Support vector machines committee classification method for computer-aided polyp detection in CT colonography. *Academic Radiology*, **12**: 479–86.

Jiang, W (2004). Process consistency for adaboost. *Annals of Statistics*, **32**(1): 13–29.

Jiang, W, R Simon (2007). A comparison of bootstrap methods and an adjusted bootstrap approach for estimating prediction error in microarray classification. *Statistics in Medicine*, **26**: 5320–34.

Jo, T, N Japkowicz (2004). A multiple resampling method for learning from imbalanced data sets. *Computational Intelligence*, **20**(1): 18–36.

Kabaila, P, H Leeb (2006). On the large-sample minimal coverage probability of confidence intervals after model selection. *Journal of the American Statistical Association*, **101**(474): 619–29.

Kendall, MG (1980). *Multivariate Analysis*. Second Edition. Charles Griffin & Company.

Kendall, M, A Stuart (1979). *The Advanced Theory of Statistics*. Volume 2, Fourth Edition. Macmillan Publishing Company.

Koltchinskii, V, B Yu (2004). Three papers on boosting: an introduction. *Annals of Statistics*, **32**(1): 12.

König, I, JD Malley, S Pajevic, C Weimar, H Diener, A Ziegler (2008). Patient-centered yes/no prognosis using learning machines. *International Journal of Data Mining and Bioinformatics*, **2**(4): 289–341.

König, I, JD Malley, C Weimar, H Diener, A Ziegler (2007). Practical experiences on the necessity of external validation. *Statistics in Medicine*, **26**(30): 5499–511.

Kooperberg, C, I Ruczinski (2005). Identifying interacting SNPs using Monte Carlo logic regression. *Genetic Epidemiology*, **28**: 157–70.

Körner, TW (2008). *Naïve Decision Making: Mathematics Applied to the Social World*. Cambridge University Press.

Kshirsagar, AM (1972). *Multivariate Analysis*. Marcel Dekker, Inc.

Kuss, O (2002). Global goodness-of-fit tests in logistic regression with sparse data. *Statistics in Medicine*, **21**: 3789–801.

Lane, T (2000). Machine learning techniques for the computer security domain of anomaly detection. PhD thesis, Purdue University, West Lafayette, IN (August 2000). Available online at: http://www.cs.unm.edu/~terran/publications.

Lawless, JF, Y Yuan (2010). Estimation of prediction error for survival models. *Statistics in Medicine*, **29**: 262–74.

Leeb, H (2005). The distribution of a linear predictor after model selection: conditional finite-sample distributions and asymptotic approximations. *Journal of Statistical Planning and Inference*, **134**: 64–89.

Leeb, H, BM Pötscher (2005). Can one estimate the unconditional distribution of the post-model-selection estimators? Online at http://mpra.ub.uni-muenchen.de/1895.

Leeb, H, BM Pötscher (2006). Can one estimate the conditional distribution of post-model-selection estimators? *Annals of Statistics*, **34**: 2554–91.

Lin, Y, Y Jeon (2006). Random forests and adaptive nearest neighbors. *Journal of the American Statistical Association*, **101**(474): 578–90.

Lippert, C, O Stegle, Z Ghahramani, KM Borgwardt (2009). A kernel method for unsupervised structured network inference. *Proceeding of the 12th International Conference on Artificial Intelligence and Statistics* (AISTATS) 2009, Clearwater Beach, Florida, USA. Vol. 5 of *Journal of Machine Learning and Research*: W&CP 5.

Lugosi, G, N Vayatis (2004). On the Bayes-risk consistency of regularized boosting methods. *Annals of Statistics*, **32**(1): 30–55.

Ma, S and J Huang (2008). Penalized feature selection and classification in bioinformatics. *Briefings in Bioinformatics*, **9**(5): 392–403.

MacKay, DJC (1992a). A practical Bayesian framework for backpropagation networks. *Neural Computation*, **4**: 448–72.

MacKay, DJC (1992b). The evidence framework applied to classification networks. *Neural Computation*, **4**: 720–36.

Mahoney, FI, D Barthel (1965). Functional evaluation: the Barthel Index. *Maryland State Medical Journal*, **14**: 56–61.

Malley, JD, AK Jerebko, MT Miller, RM Summers (2003). Variance reduction for error estimation when classifying colon polyps from CT colonography. Medical Imaging 2003: Physiology and Function: Methods, Systems, and Applications (AV Clough, AA Amini, Eds). *Proceedings of SPIE*, **5031**: 570–78.

Mease, D, A Wyner (2008). Evidence contrary to the statistical view of boosting. *Journal of Machine Leaning and Research*, **9**: 131–56; Response and Rejoinder: 157–201.

Mease, D, AJ Wyner, A Buja (2007). Boosted classification trees and class probability/quantile estimation. *Journal of Machine Leaning and Research*, **8**: 409–39.

Meinshausen, N (2006). Quantile regression forests. *Journal of Machine Learning Research*, **7**: 983–99.

Melnik, O, Y Vardi, C-H Zhang (2007). Concave learners for Rankboost. *Journal of Machine Learning Research*, **8**: 791–812.

Melvin, I, E Ie, J Weston, WS Noble, C Leslie (2007). Multi-class protein classification using adaptive codes. *Journal of Machine Learning Research*, **8**: 1557–81.

Mielke, PW Jr, KJ Berry (2001). *Permutation Methods: A Distance Function Approach.* Springer-Verlag.

Miller, MT, AK Jerebko, JD Malley, RM Summers (2003). Feature selection for computer-aided polyp detection using genetic algorithms. Medical Imaging 2003: Physiology and Function: Methods, Systems, and Applications (AV Clough, AA Amini, Eds), *Proceedings of SPIE*, **5031**: 102–10.

Miller, ME, CD Langefeld, WM Tierney, SL Hui, CJ McDonald (1993). Validation of probabilistic predictions. *Medical Decision Making*, **13**(1): 49–57.

Minku, FL, TB Ludermir (2008). Clustering and co-evolution to construct neural network ensembles: an experimental study. *Neural Networks*, **21**: 1363–79.

Mojirsheibani, M (1999). Combining classifiers via discretization. *Journal of the American Statistical Association*, **94**: 600–609.

Mojirsheibani, M (2002). An almost surely optimal combined classification rule. *Journal of Multivariate Analysis*, **81**: 28–46.

Molinaro, A, R Simon, R Pfeiffer (2005). Prediction error estimation: a comparison of resampling methods. *Bioinformatics*, **21**: 3301–7.

Montori, VM, GH Guyatt (2008). Progress in evidence-based medicine. *Journal of the American Medical Association*, **300**(15): 1814–16.

Moons, KGM, ART Donders, EW Steyerberg, FE Harrell (2004). Penalized maximum likelihood estimation to directly adjust diagnostic and prognostic prediction models for overoptimism: a clinical example. *Journal of Clinical Epidemiology*, **57**: 1262–70.

Muirhead, RJ (1982). *Aspects of Multivariate Statistical Theory*. John Wiley & Sons.

Mukhopadhyay, N (2009). Letter to the Editor. *American Statistician*, **63**(1): 102–3.

Newcombe, RG (1998a). Improved confidence intervals for the difference between binomial proportions based on paired data. *Statistics in Medicine*, **17**: 2635 –50.

Newcombe, RG (1998b). Two-sided confidence intervals for the single proportion: comparison of seven methods. *Statistics in Medicine*, **17**: 857–72.

Newcombe, RG (1998c). Interval estimation for the difference between independent proportions. *Statistics in Medicine*, **17**: 873–90.

Newcombe, RG (2006a). Confidence intervals for an effect size measure based on the Mann–Whitney statistic. Part 1: General issues and tail area based methods. *Statistics in Medicine*, **25**(4): 543–57.

Newcombe, RG (2006b). Confidence intervals for an effect size measure based on the Mann–Whitney statistic. Part 2: Asymptotic methods and evaluation. *Statistics in Medicine*, **25**(4): 559–73.

Newcombe, RG (2007). Comments on "Confidence intervals for a ratio of binomial proportions based on paired data." *Statistics in Medicine*, **26**(25): 4684–5.

Nicodemus, K, JD Malley (2009). Predictor correlation impacts machine learning algorithms: implications for genomic studies. *Bioinformatics*, **25**(15): 1884–90.

Nicodemus, KK, JD Malley, C Strobl, A Ziegler (2010). The behaviour of random forest permutation-based variable importance measures under predictor correlation. *BMC Bioinformatics*, **11**: 110–23.

Omurlu, IK, M Ture, F Tokatli (2009). The comparisons of random survival forests and Cox regression analysis with simulation and an application related to breast cancer. *Expert Systems with Applications*, **36**: 8582–8588.

Ottenbacher, KJ, HR Ottenbacher, L Tooth, GV Ostir (2004). A review of two journals found that articles using multivariable logistic regression frequently did not report commonly recommended assumptions. *Journal of Clinical Epidemiology*, **57**: 1147–52.

Ottenbacher, KJ, PM Smith, SB Illig, RT Linn, RC Fiedler, CV Granger (2001). Comparison of logistic regression and neural networks to predict rehospitalization in patients with stroke. *Journal of Clinical Epidemiology*, **54**: 1159–65.

Pace, L, A Salvan (1997). *Principles of Statistical Inference*. World Scientific.

Pepe, MS (2003). *The Statistical Evaluation of Medical Tests for Classification and Prediction*. Oxford University Press.

Potter, DM (2005). A permutation test for inference in logistic regression with small- and moderate-sized data sets. *Statistics in Medicine*, **24**: 693–708.

Potter, DM (2008). Notes for CRAN Library package "logregperm." Inference in Logistic Regression. Date/Publication 2008–04–22 07:36:27.

Predd, J, R Seiringer, EH Lieb, D Osherson, V Poor, S Kulkarni (2009). Probabilistic coherence and proper scoring rules. *IEEE Transactions on Information Theory*, in press.

Ramsay, JO, BW Silverman (1997). *Functional Data Analysis*. Springer-Verlag.

Ratkowsky, DA (1990). *Handbook of Nonlinear Regression Models*. Marcel Dekker.

Rogers, W, T Wagner (1978). A finite sample distribution-free performance bound for local discrimination rules. *Annals of Statistics*, **6**: 506–14.

Ruczinski, I, C Kooperberg, ML LeBlanc (2003). Logic regression. *Journal of Computational and Graphical Statistics*, **12**(3): 475–511.

Rutjes, AWS, JB Reitsma, M Di Nisio, N Smidt, JC van Rijn, PMM Bossuyt (2006). Evidence of bias and variation in diagnostic accuracy studies. *Canadian Medical Association Journal*, **174**(4): 1–12 (online).

Saari, DG (1995). A chaotic exploration of aggregation paradoxes. *SIAM Review*, **37**(1): 37–52.

Saari, DG (2008). *Disposing Dictators, Demystifying Voting Paradoxes: Social Choice Analysis*. Cambridge University Press.

Sabato, S, S Shalev-Shwartz (2008). Ranking categorical features using generalization properties. *Journal of Machine Learning Research*, **9**: 1083–14.

Schölkopf, B, AJ Smola (2002). *Learning with Kernels: Support Vector Machines, Regularization, Optimization, and Beyond*. MIT Press.

Schölkopf, B, R Herbrich, AJ Smola, RC Williamson (2001). A generalized representer theorem. Proceedings of the 14th Annual Conference on Computational Learning Theory, COLT 2001. *Lecture Notes in Computer Science* (Springer): 416–26.

Schwarz, DF, IR König, A Ziegler (2010). On safari to Random Jungle: a fast implementation of Random Forests for high dimensional data. *Bioinformatics*, in press.

Seber, GAF, CJ Wild (1989). *Nonlinear Regression*. John Wiley & Sons.

Severini, TA (2000). *Likelihood Methods in Statistics*. Oxford University Press.

Shao, H, LC Burrage, DS Sinasac, AE Hill, SR Ernest, W O'Brien, HW Courtland, KJ Jepsen, A Kirby, EJ Kulbokas, MJ Daly, KW Broman, ES Lander, JH Nadeau (2008). Genetic architecture of complex traits: large phenotypic effects and pervasive epistasis. *Proceedings of the National Academy of Science USA*, **105**(50): 19910–4.

Shapire, RE, Y Singer (2000). BoosTexter: a boosting-based system for text categorization. *Machine Learning*, **39**(2/3): 135–68.

Shi, T, D Seligson, AS Belldebrun, A Palotie, S Horvath (2005). Tumor classification by tissue microarray profiling: random forest clustering applied to renal cell carcinoma. *Modern Biology*, **18**: 547–57.

Shieh, G (2001). The inequality between the coefficient of determination and the sum of squared simple correlation coefficients. *The American Statistician*, **55**(2): 121–4.

Spanos, A (2010). The discovery of argon: a case for learning from data? *Philosophy of Science*, **77**(3): 359–80.

Spiegelhalter, DJ, EC Marshall (2006). Strategies for inference robustness in focused modelling. *Journal of Applied Statistics*, **33**(2): 217–31.

Sprent, P, NC Smeeton (2001). *Applied Nonparametric Statistical Methods*. Third Edition. Chapman & Hall/CRC Press.

Steinwart, I (2005). Consistency of support vector machines and other regularized kernel classifiers. *IEEE Transactions on Information Theory*, **51**(1): 128–42.

Steyerberg, EW, GJJM Borsboom, HC van Houwelingen, MJC Eijkemans, JDF Habbema (2004). Validation and updating of predictive logistic regression models: a study on sample size and shrinkage. *Statistics in Medicine*, **23**: 2567–86.

Strobl, C, JD Malley, G Tutz (2009). An introduction to recursive partitioning: rationale, application, and characteristics of classification and regression trees, bagging, and random forests. *Psychological Methods*, **14**(4): 323–48.

Stone, C (1977). Consistent nonparametric regression. *Annals of Statistics*, **13**: 689–705.

Strobl, C, A-L Boulesteix, T Kneib, T Augustin, A Zeileis (2008). Conditional variable importance for random forests. *BMC Bioinformatics*, **9**: 307–18.

Strobl C, A-L Boulesteix, A Zeileis, T Hothorn (2007). Bias in random forest variable importance measures: illustrations, sources and a solution. *BMC Bioinformatics*, **8**: 25–46.

Tango, T (1998). Equivalence test and confidence interval for the difference in proportions for the paired-sample design. *Statistics in Medicine*, **17**: 891–908.

Tango, T (1999). Improved confidence intervals for the difference between binomial proportions based on paired data (with Author's Reply). *Statititics in Medicine*, **18**: 3511–13.

Tango, T (2000). Confidence intervals for differences in correlated binary proportions (with Author's Reply). *Statistics in Medicine*, **19**: 133–9.

Tibshirani, R (1996). Regression shrinkage and selection via the lasso. *Journal of the Royal Statistical Society*, Series B, **58**(1): 267–88.

Toussaint, GT (1971). Note on optimal selection of independent binary-valued features for pattern recognition. *IEEE Transactions on Information Theory*, **17**: 618.

Twisk, JWR (2006). *Applied Multilevel Analysis*. Cambridge University Press.

Übeyli, ED (2006). Combining neural network models for automated diagnostic systems. *Journal of Medical Systems*, **30**: 483–8.

Vapnik, V (2000). *The Nature of Statistical Learning Theory*. Second Edition. Springer-Verlag.

Varma, S, R Simon (2006). Bias in error estimation when using cross-validation for model selection. *BMC Bioinformatics*, **7**: 91–8.

Walker, JA, JF Miller (2008). The automatic acquisition, evolution and reuse of modules in cartesian genetic programming. *IEEE Transactions on Evolutionary Computation*, **12**(4): 397–417.

Wang, BX, N Japkowicz (2008). Boosting support vector machines for imbalanced data sets. *Proceedings of the 17th International Symposium on Methodologies for Intelligent Systems* (ISMIS 2008).

Ward, MM, MR Hendrey, JD Malley, TJ Learch, JC Davis Jr, JD Reveille, MH Weisman (2009). Clinical and immunogenetic prognostic factors for radiographic severity in ankylosing spondylitis. *Arthritis & Rheumatism (Arthritis Care & Research)*, **61**(7): 859–66.

Ward, MM, S Pajevic, J Dreyfuss, JD Malley (2006). Short-term prediction of mortality in patients with systemic lupus erythematosus: classification of outcomes using random forests. *Arthritis & Rheumatism (Arthritis Care & Research)*, **55**(1): 74–80.

Welsh, AH (1996). *Aspects of Statistical Inference.* John Wiley & Sons.

Willan, AR, EM Pinto (2005). The value of information and optimal clinical trial design. *Statistics in Medicine*, **24**: 1791–806.

Willett, JB, JD Singer (1988). Another cautionary note about R^2: its use in weighted least-square regression analysis. *American Statistician*, **42**(3): 236–8.

Wolpert, DH (1992). Stacked generalization. *Neural Networks*, **5**: 241–59.

Wolpert, DH, WG Macready (1996). Combining stacking with bagging to improve a learning algorithm. Santa Fe Institute technical report, August 1996, SFI-TR-96–03–123.

Zakai, A, Y Ritov (2008). How local should a learning method be? *21st Annual Conference on Learning Theory (COLT)*: 205–16.

Zakai, A, Y Ritov (2009). Consistency and localizability. *Journal of Machine Learning Research*, **10**: 827–56.

Zhang, T (2004a). Statistical behavior and consistency of classification methods based on convex risk minimization. *Annals of Statistics*, **32**(1): 56–134.

Zhang, H (2004b). The optimality of naive Bayes. *Proceedings of the 17th International FLAIRS (Florida Artificial Intelligence Research Society) Conference.* Association for the Advancement of Artificial Intelligence Press.

Zhao, Z, H Liu (2007). Searching for interacting features. *Proceedings of the International Joint Conference on Artificial Intelligence*: 1156–61.

Zhou, X-H, G Qin (2003). A new confidence interval for the difference between two binomial proportions of paired data. Technical Report No. 205, University of Washington.

Zhou, X-H, NA Obuchowski, DK McClish (2002). *Statistical Methods in Diagnostic Medicine.* John Wiley & Sons.

Index

%GOFLOGIT SAS macro
for goodness-of-fit 12, 103
632+ method 207
accuracy 95, 114, 117, 134, 215
Agresti, Alan 10
Akaike information criterion 22
analysis of covariance 170
analysis of variance 10, 124
artificial neural networks 53

backward stepwise elimination
181, 182
balancing 82
Barthel Index 62
base classifier 54
Bayes classifiers 45
Bayes consistency 31, 32, 33, 34, 50, 152,
253, 256
Bayes error 222
Bayes optimal decision rule 38
Bayes risk 32
Bayesian information criterion 22
Bayesian model averaging 251
beer consumption example 176
benchmarking 32, 56
bias 109, 220, 226, 233
bimodal 183
Boltzmann learning machines 29
BoosTexter 77
boosting 12, 34, 38, 54, 68, 70, 74, 84

bootstrap resampling 65, 112, 134, 137,
198, 202, 218, 227
Breiman, Leo 10, 137

C language 12
calibration 106, 107, 112
cardiac functioning example 173
case-to-case distance 211, 213
cell cultures experiment 207
cholesterol study example 11, 58, 66, 94,
107, 165, 228
classification 14, 50, 113, 240
classification tree 22
classifier 225, 251
clustering 17, 143, 261
coefficient of determination 177, 193
coefficients 93, 101, 180
committee 34, 117, 249, 250
composite clinical score 9
conditional inference forest 10, 13, 154
conditional probability 45, 46
confidence interval 11, 108, 215, 234
confusion matrix 217
constraints 21
continuous outcomes 9, 36, 239
convergence 101
correlation 10, 44, 101, 115, 136,
157, 165, 168, 177, 201, 216,
234, 248
correlation coefficient 158, 161

crop yield 174
cross-validation 112, 198, 222, 224
cubic histogram 34
Cutler, Adele 10, 137

data integrity 231
data mining 15, 185
decision boundary 52, 59, 66, 87, 98, 102,
    125, 133
decision rule 94, 95, 102, 129, 132
decision trees 10, 29, 67, 84, 112,
    118, 120
dependent variable 16
Devroye, Luc (DGL) 14
discriminant analysis 37
discriminant function 43
distance function 143
distance measure 49
down-sampling 142, 219
dropping down a tree 118

empirical risk minimization 225
ensemble methods 57, 117, 247, 249
error estimation 217, 219, 221, 226, 232
error rate 64, 67, 70, 71, 74, 76, 94, 113,
    141, 198, 223, 248
Euclidean distance 49, 143, 211
evolutionary algorithm 55
evolutionary computing 29

false negative 67
false positive 67
Farrington statistic 104
features (variables) 16, 47, 62, 70, 74,
    112, 114, 120, 132, 137, 153, 212
functional data estimation 203

gene expression transcripts 17
generalized additive model 44, 53
genetic algorithm 55

Gini concentration measure 105
Gini error 140
Gini index 124, 133
goodness-of-fit 92, 103, 116
group prediction 43

hidden layer 53
high-order correlation 8
Hopfield neural networks 29
Hosmer–Lemeshow test 104
Hothorn, Torsten 13

image classification 260
imbalanced data 63, 205
important features (variables) 7
independence 229, 248
independent variable 16
interactions 7, 92, 95, 99, 132
interpretable model 7

k-nearest neighbor 22, 34, 48, 68, 72, 76,
    83, 220
kernel functions 69
kernel methods 29, 50, 51
knowledge discovery 15
Kruskal–Wallis 189
König, Inke 11

lasso 21
layered nearest neighbor 152
learning machine 14, 60, 70, 115, 130, 137,
    224, 234, 249
leave-one-out method 198, 226, 241
likelihood function 22, 100
linear discriminant 31, 43, 66, 80, 83, 115,
    228, 242
linear model 53, 56
linear regression 4, 22, 37, 41, 53, 157
linear support vector machine 51
local 35, 49, 52, 67, 73, 128, 162, 256

logic regression 16, 47, 51
logistic regression 4, 11, 25, 27, 42, 66, 91,
    106, 114
logitboost 27, 38, 55
longitudinal data 260
lupus (SLE) study example 9, 11, 61, 70,
    79, 81, 112, 129

machine learning 15
Mahalanobis distance 242
matched case-control
MatLab 12
mean squared error 240
merging models 186
misclassification 67, 97, 141, 205, 237
missing data 9
model averaging 196
model richness 22, 53, 128
Mojirsheibani, Majid 252
Monte Carlo 87, 213, 231
multidimensional scaling (MDS)
    18, 143
multilevel models 170
multiple models 186
multiple response permutation
    procedures (MRPP) 210
mXCV cross-validation 223

naïve Bayes machine 26, 46, 201
nearest neighbors 34
neighborhood 49, 52, 256
neural networks 29, 39, 53, 68, 71,
    76, 83
Newcombe, Robert 11
node 120, 140
node purity 133
nonlinear model 53
nonparametric 16, 22
nonparametric density estimation 203
null hypothesis 209, 214

Occam's Razor 187
optimization 79, 69
out-of-bag (OOB) sampling 65, 71, 79,
    134, 137, 218, 227, 232
outcome 14, 63
outliers 44, 159, 166
overall error rate 64, 65, 217
overfitting 21, 54, 128, 130
oversampling 206

parameter 92
parametric bootstrap methods 203
partial correlation 175
pattern recognition 15
Pearson statistic 104
penalized maximum likelihood 112
performance 65, 74, 80, 215, 228
permutation procedure for testing group
    differences 210
permutation tests 207
pooling lists 186
pooling machines 251, 252
population incidence 219
precision 64, 217
prediction 14, 54, 58, 92, 118, 222,
    236, 256
prediction engine 4, 15, 117, 213,
    225, 248
predictive accuracy 11
predictors 16, 43, 47, 61, 62, 63, 70, 143,
    178, 247
principal components analysis 19
priors 45
probabilistic learning theory 5
probabilistic pattern recognition 49
probability 92, 248
probability estimates 102
probability function 22
probability of group membership 43, 45,
    92, 103, 106, 113, 128

Proc IML 12
Proc Logistic 12
proximity 19
pruning 128, 138
purity 122, 123

quadratic discriminant function 44

R language 12
R-squared 105, 177, 193
Random Forests 10, 12, 26, 34,
  50, 62, 63, 75, 77, 112, , 116,
  137, 152
Random Jungles 10, 13, 34, 50, 112, 116,
  152, 153, 214
randomization 223
ranking features (variables) 86
rate of convergence 31
ratio sampling 219
receiver operator curves 103
reference model 113
regression 4, 239
regression tree 163
repeated measures 260
resampling 111, 112, 198, 218,
  225, 227
robustness of the inference 169
ROC curves 236
rotation method 240

sample size 8, 136, 142, 204, 251
sample variance 124, 223
sampling with replacement 199, 218
SAS 12
Schwarz, Daniel 13
sensitivity 64, 68, 81, 84, 94, 114, 141, 205,
  217, 231, 236
sequential scheme 34
shrinkage methods 112
Simpson's paradox 170

simulated annealing 29
simulated data 8
simulated study 58
single nucleotide polymorphisms (SNPs)
  7, 17, 46, 136, 231
small sample sizes 206
software 12
sparse 104
specificity 64, 82, 84, 94, 114, 205, 217,
  231, 236
spinal curvature example 172, 184
splitting 120
splitting to purity 35, 152
stacking 117
statistically balanced blocks 34
stepwise regression 181
stopping rules 127
stroke study example 11, 62, 75, 79, 103,
  144, 234
structural risk minimization 225
subsets 9
super classifiers 32, 57, 79
supervised learning 17, 144
support vector machine (SVM) 11, 16, 33,
  44, 50, 69, 83
support vectors 52
survival 15, 62
survival forest 259
survival machines 259
SVMLight 12
systemic lupus erythematosus (SLE) 61

Tango, Toshiro 11, 257
terminal node 119, 130, 143,
  152, 253
testing 60
thresholds 58, 95, 237
total balancing 219
training 60, 77, 100, 121, 134, 224,
  226, 229

transfer function 53
transition node 119
tree complexity 128, 138
tuning 70, 141, 257
two-fold cross-validation (2XCV) 222

unbalanced 63, 82, 94
unbalanced bootstrap sampling 205
unbalanced data 205, 218,
   231, 233
unbalanced groups 8
under-sampling 142, 219
unequal group sizes 212, 218

unequal variances 101
unsupervised learning 17, 37, 144

validation 6, 149
Vapnik–Chernovenkis dimension
   23, 54, 128
variable importance 116, 132
variable permutation 134
variable selection 102
vitamin E experiment 207

Ward, Michael 11
Wilcoxon rank sum test 237

Printed in the United States
by Baker & Taylor Publisher Services